1001
WAYS TO
get in shape

Susannah
Marriott

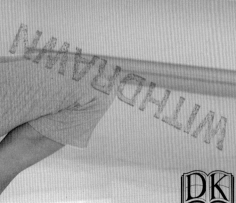

DK

P9-AGO-415

LONDON, NEW YORK, MUNICH,
MELBOURNE, DELHI

For my daughters

Project editor Angela Baynham
Design Carole Ash at Project 360
Senior editor Helen Murray
Senior art editor Sarah Ponder
Design assistant Charlotte Seymour
US editors Shannon Beatty and Christy Lusiak
Photographer Ruth Jenkinson
Creative technical support Sonia Charbonnier
Production editor Ben Marcus
Production controller Hema Gohil
Managing editors Esther Ripley and Penny Warren
Managing art editor Marianne Markham
Jacket designer Charlotte Seymour
Category publisher Peggy Vance
Yoga tips Amanda Brown
Homeopathic/herbal tips Julia Linfoot BSc MCPH RSHom

Caution: The tips in this book are intended for healthy adults. It's best to seek the advice of your doctor before beginning a weight-loss regime, especially if you are pregnant, breastfeeding, or have any medical condition. Do not calorie-control a child's or teenager's diet without first consulting a doctor. Also consult your doctor before starting an exercise program if you are over 35, overweight, haven't exercised in a long time, are pregnant, have recently given birth, or have any medical condition. If you are pregnant or have a medical condition, do not use herbs (including herbal teas) without consulting a qualified herbal practitioner. Use only the essential oils specified and never use more drops than recommended. See cautions on individual tips and recipes. The advice and information on health matters given in this book is not intended as a substitute for qualified medical advice and neither the publisher nor the author accept any legal responsibility for personal injury or damage or loss arising from its use or misuse.

First American edition, 2009

Published in the United States by
DK Publishing
375 Hudson Street
New York, New York 10014

09 10 11 10 9 8 7 6 5 4 3 2
AD405—February 2009

Published in Great Britain by Dorling Kindersley Limited

A catalog record for this book is available from the Library of Congress.

ISBN 978-0-7566-4204-4

DK books are available at special discounts when purchased in bulk for sales promotions, premiums, fund-raising, or educational use. For details, contact: DK Publishing Special Markets, 375 Hudson Street, New York, New York 10014 or SpecialSales@dk.com.

Color reproduction by MDP, UK

Printed and bound in China by Sheck Wah Tong

Discover more at
www.dk.com

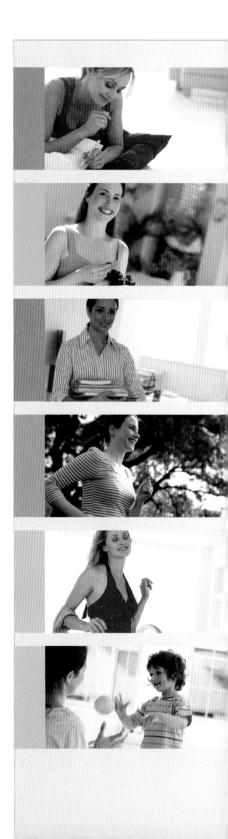

Contents

Introduction

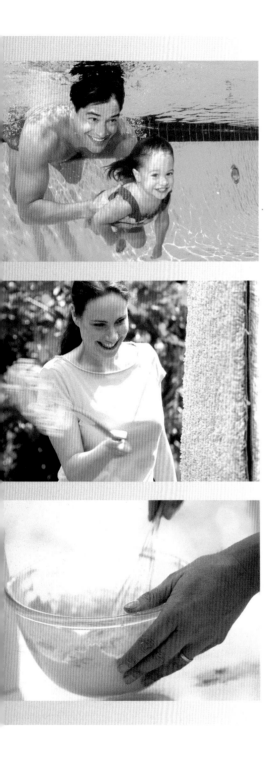

Modern living makes it incredibly difficult for us to get—and stay—in shape. With the advent of processed food and supersized portions, the average American now consumes around 200 calories more each day than in the 1970s. And we don't burn off calories like we used to either, thanks to labor-saving devices such as ready-made meals, sedentary screen-based jobs, and a long-hours work culture, and because we prefer TV viewing over more active leisure pursuits. In the US, two-thirds of adults are overweight and more than a third of these are obese; in the UK (Europe's weight-problem leader), a quarter of adults will be clinically obese by 2010. Obesity ranks second only to smoking as a preventable cause of premature death, and one study found that obese people have a higher risk of depression, while children deprived of enough activity or family mealtimes seem to fail to thrive intellectually, emotionally, and socially.

How do we counteract obesity?

How do we break out of this? The answer is much simpler and more accessible than enduring intense sessions at the gym—just be a little more active every day, cook meals from raw ingredients, and eat them at home with family or friends (and turn off the TV). Indeed, what burns most calories, found Maastricht University research in the Netherlands, is not short, intense gym sessions, but upping your activity levels so that you are moderately active for longer most days: park a little further from the store; wash, chop, and stir as you cook; weed a vegetable patch; and stand rather than sit. As well as keeping us looking shapely by toning muscles, oiling the joints, and improving posture and coordination, being more active keeps us holistically in better shape, reducing risk of heart disease, type-2 diabetes, cancers of the breast and colon, stroke, high blood pressure, and osteoporosis.

What role does food play?

To lose weight and keep it off, it's important to change the way you eat permanently—and this isn't a chore if you allow yourself to be seduced by the pleasure of real food. In fact, it feels positively indulgent, and this is why it works. If the foods on our plates are processed, obesity and chronic disease follow, according to the World Health Organization, because these products tend to be loaded with fat, sugar, salt, and calories, and are often low in nutrients. If your plate is piled with unprocessed foods—mostly vegetables, fruit, pulses, and whole grains, with smaller amounts of meat, fish, and low-fat dairy produce—it's hard not to shed excess pounds, maintain a healthy weight, and effortlessly shape up every part of your body and mind. Not only that, your taste buds and senses wake up. Cram your food cart, pantry, refrigerator, and garden with foods that are naturally rich in color and intense in flavor—foods that look like they did growing in the field or ocean or on the tree. When everyday food becomes delicious and your body feels light and energized, you won't get hung up on what not to eat or the latest superfoods, and you will crave the foods that keep you in shape forever.

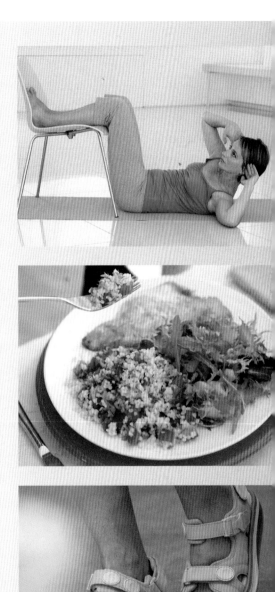

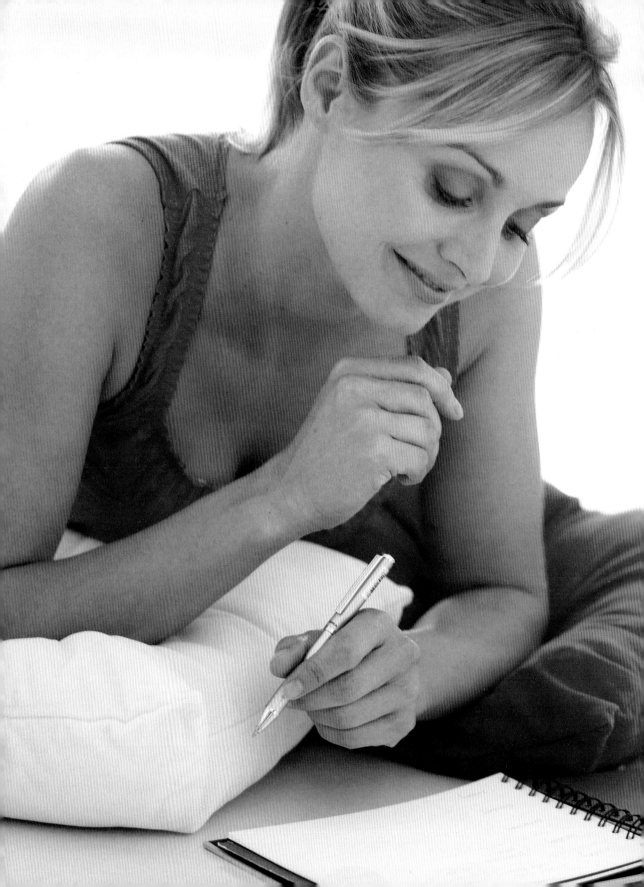

1 Think yourself in shape

Many people think that fitness begins in the gym. However, research suggests that it starts much nearer to home—in your head. It is only by igniting and maintaining your motivation to make some real changes in your life—to become more active and to eat more healthily—that you will achieve your fitness goals. The trick is to find ways to enjoy exercise and discover the pleasures of good eating: once you fall in love with real food and the buzz you get from exercising you'll never want to give them up, and that's the best way to stay in shape forever. In this first chapter you'll find ways to set realistic and achievable aims, to counter cravings, maintain motivation, and above all to boost the amount of pleasure you enjoy in your life.

Great expectations

To start thinking yourself in shape, stand back and take a look at where you are now and where you'd like to get to. Don't worry if you've tried to get fit or lose weight in the past but have given up, there are easy ways to change your perception of yourself so that you start to feel and act like a winner. Release your imagination, focus on keeping your mind in a positive frame, then be clear about your goals and try not to give up before you have achieved them.

1
You've already begun
By reading this far you've already started to lead a more healthy life; congratulate yourself. Research has found that people who tell themselves they are healthy and active tend to maintain a healthy lifestyle long term.

2
Use your imagination
Close your eyes and imagine yourself pounding effortlessly along a beautiful beach—smell the ozone, sense the endorphins coursing through your body, feel the breeze cooling your brow, imagine your heart beating strongly and your lungs expanding. If you can feel this good just thinking about it, you are already on your way to being an active person.

3
Assess your aims
What did you want to achieve when you bought this book? Write down your answer. Make your aims specific: not just to lose weight or get fitter, but to get into last year's bikini, tone your upper arms, or eat more vegetables. Set yourself a time line for achieving each goal. Research at Aberdeen University in Scotland found that people who set specific goals lost significantly more weight than people who were vague about their aims.

4
Think positive
Use active verbs and positive words to describe your goals: "I will eat more healthily" rather than "I'd benefit from losing a few pounds." Saying what you're going to do fixes the intention more effectively in your unconscious mind and dispels negative thinking.

5
Mantra for the day
Set yourself an objective and repeat it over and over. For example, "Today I will stand rather than sit; walk rather than stand; jog rather than walk; and run rather than jog."

6
Watch your waistband
Look at where you put on weight. Fat deposited around the abdomen is especially hazardous to health, so when your waistband gets tight, it's time to act.

7
Waist to hip ratio
The relationship of your waist to your hips is a good indicator of whether your heart is in good shape. Measure around the narrowest part of your waist, then the widest part of your hips and buttocks. Use a calculator to divide the waist measurement by the hip measurement. For women, having an answer of more than 0.8 increases the risk of cardiovascular disease and diabetes (for men, the ratio is more than 1).

8

Find your BMI

Your body mass index (BMI) may be a useful guide to whether you need to lose weight. Divide your weight in kilos by your height in meters (squared) or use an online BMI calculator (see www.bdaweightwise.com). If you have a reading over 25, you'll benefit from losing weight; if it's over 30 you're classed as overweight and at risk of health problems. If your reading is over 35, you should visit your doctor.

9

Use a fitness planner

Plan out fitness targets. Allocate specific activities to specific days: 30 minutes on the treadmill, a lunchtime walk, football with the kids. Next to each one, write down what you need to do beforehand: book a class, wash your workout gear, call your fitness buddy. Leave space to record what you actually did and to describe your post-workout sensations and energy levels.

10

Keep a food diary

Start a food diary with three columns: what you ate; where you

Free your imagination— envision yourself running along a beautiful beach and savor the sensations.

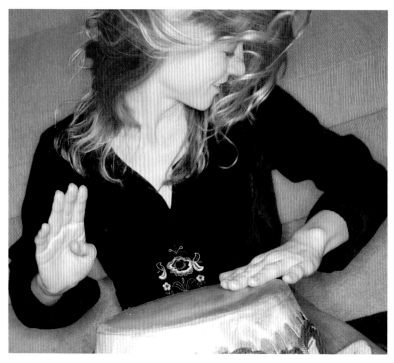

Build brisk activity into your day doing anything from vigorous cleaning to playing drums.

12

Consider your age

As you age, you require fewer calories per day: in your 30s and 40s you need 200 less than you did in your 20s; once you hit your 50s, cut another 200 if you want to stay in shape.

13

Write your future

If you enjoy writing, take time out to write about your life as you live it. As an introduction, describe your everyday life now: who you are, what you do, the people around you, and what you would like to change. Be candid! Then see if you can plot out 12 chapters, one for each of the next 12 months. Think about the things you would like to happen and the obstacles you need to overcome, then build them into your story. Post it as a blog—you might even gain publisher interest...

Put it in writing: describe your life now, then devise a plot for the way you might like the next 12 months to unfold.

ate and with whom; how you felt after you had eaten. After a week, look back at the patterns. Do you eat less healthily when watching TV or when you are out with friends? Where and when do you eat most healthily? What would it take to replicate healthy patterns? In one study it was revealed that people who used food diaries ate around 15 percent less than those who kept no record of what they ate.

five days a week. If you're already doing this, gradually build up to 60 minutes. You can break it down into 10–15 minute bursts, and you don't have to do it at the gym: activities such as vigorous cleaning, walking up a hill carrying the groceries, or practicing the drums all count toward your total.

11

Know what you need

To keep the body in shape we need to incorporate at least 30 minutes of brisk activity into our day at least

Keep it real

Expecting to achieve an overnight transformation in lifestyle or body shape sets you up for failure. Successful people are more realistic, making only small changes, but ones they can maintain every day and build into a lasting lifestyle overhaul. Your long-term goal might simply be to stay the weight you are right now, or to tone up your muscles so they take on a more pleasing shape.

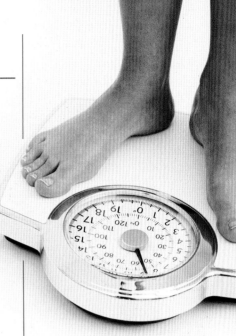

14
Weight expectations
For long-lasting weight loss, don't cut your body weight by more than 5–10 percent over the next six months. This is a realistic amount for most to manage and maintain.

15
Little by little
The healthiest amount of weight to lose is no more than 1lb (450g) a week. Do this by eating 500–600 calories fewer than your energy needs every day. For an average woman, that means 1,500 calories daily; men are permitted 300 more.

16
Halt weight gain
One study estimated that cutting out 100 calories a day would halt weight gain (most of us gain around 2lb/900g a year). You can do this by simply eating one less cookie a day.

17
Stat fear
Numbers are neutral—repeat this before you weigh or measure yourself. If they make you feel sad or angry or you find them intimidating, forget weights and measurements and gauge your body shape by how your clothes fit, how you feel, and

Get on the scale only on set days at set intervals as far apart as you can manage.

the amount of energy you have. You don't need the scale to tell you if you have gained weight.

18
Think long term
Don't weigh yourself every day. Do it once a week or every two weeks—or less often—to encourage long-term positive thinking. If you choose to have your percentage of body fat measured, don't do this more often than once a month. But do remember to fill in your fitness and food journals every day: this type of self-monitoring encourages you to keep making healthy choices.

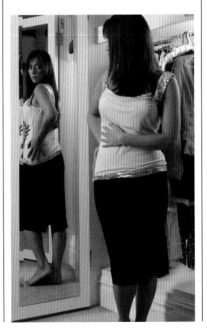

If you prefer, forget weights and measurements and focus on fit and feel.

Taking a brisk jog at lunchtime will set you on the road to fitness.

19
Keep notes
Carry around a small notebook or use your electronic organizer to track every bite you take, ready to transfer to your food journal.

20
Easy does it
If your doctor has classified you as obese, don't panic—even moderate weight loss reduces your risk of heart disease and diabetes and can lower cholesterol levels and blood pressure.

21
Mini-goals
Once you have an overall goal, work back from it, setting up a roadmap of realistic mini-goals that steer you to your end point. Write them down, making sure that they are positive and practical—order a weekly produce box, clear the freezer of junk food, get your bike serviced, make soup for Monday lunch—and then set times to achieve each one.

22
Think every day
The little things you manage to do every day, such as leaving the cookie jar empty or taking a lunchtime jog, lead to success.

23
Consult the experts
If you prefer being told what to do by an expert, find an online calorie-counting program that gives specific counts for food portions and sets out what you need at each meal. Try the American Dietetic Association's at www.eatright.org.

24
The 80-20 rule
Accept that you're human and that we are all imperfect. As long as you keep to your diet and fitness regime 80 percent of the time, you can forgive yourself the 20 percent of times that you lapse.

Pleasure not pain

The least successful diet plans leave us feeling deprived. It's hard to stick to deprivation diets because we're hardwired to choose pleasure over pain. However, if you embrace real food—the kind you cook at home using fresh, tasty ingredients—you will discover a diet you'll look forward to eating for the rest of your life.

25
Forget dieting
A 2007 study into temporary diets found that most dieters regained any weight they lost. Yo-yo dieting has also been linked to reduced immunity, high blood pressure, and exponential weight gain.

26
Ditch the scale
The University of Minnesota School of Public Health found that the frequency with which teenage girls weighed themselves correlated with increased bingeing and other unhealthy strategies, such as missing meals, vomiting, or taking diet pills. Over five years, girls who weighed themselves often gained nearly twice as much weight as those who didn't.

27
Let go with flowers
Rock Water is a lesser-known Bach Flower Essence and suits people who are hard on themselves and don't let go or have fun. If you make strict rules for yourself around food, this essence could help you to understand that inner harmony is more powerful than externally enforced behaviour. Place 4 drops in water and sip.

28
Strive for balance
Eating well means eating something from each of the food groups at mealtimes: fruit and vegetables; grains and potatoes; meat, fish, or veggie alternatives; dairy produce; and fatty, sugary foods. Make fruit and vegetables one third of your plate and grains or potatoes another third. That leaves the last third for meat or fish, dairy produce, and a little fatty or sugary food as a treat.

29
Eat more!
Excluding foods from your diet risks nutrient deficiency. It's better to think of dieting as a chance to boost the number of foods (and nutrients) you consume every day. Add in as many different fruits and vegetables as you can (9–13 portions if possible): as well as being nutrient-rich, they are packed with filling water and fiber, leaving less room for the foods associated with obesity (saturated fat and sugar).

30
Don't starve
Hunger makes us reach for calorie-rich foods. To stave off hunger, have three moderate meals a day plus healthy snacks (eat something every three hours). A South African study found that men who ate a small breakfast followed by healthy morning snacks ate almost 30 percent fewer calories at lunch.

Eating plenty of healthy food is more likely to result in weight loss than not eating at all.

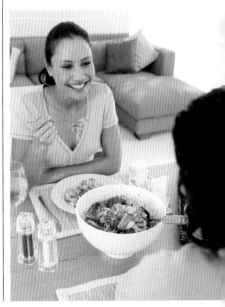

31

Eat until you're full

Start noticing the difference between feeling sated and feeling stuffed. See if you can stop eating at the point at which you feel pleasantly full, but not uncomfortable or sleepy.

32

Feel the hunger

What does hunger feel like? Can you distinguish it from boredom or expectation? Spend a day not eating until your stomach, rather than your mind, feels empty.

33

Sit down to eat

Thinking of food as something to savor and a form of relaxation rather than an opportunity to refuel can stop you from taking in unnoticed calories as you graze on the run. To make mealtimes special, stop work, turn off the TV, set the table and sit down to eat—preferably with a knife and fork and your food on a plate!

34

Eat mindfully

Be aware of everything you put in your mouth. Is it delicious? Do you really want to eat it? Does it make you feel good? If you answer no to any of these questions, keep your mouth shut.

35

Cancel the gym

If a gym membership is a constant source of stress or guilt, cancel it and find more lifestyle-friendly ways to exercise, perhaps biking to work twice a week or gardening.

36

Make time for treats

Make a list of all the physical activities that make you feel good about yourself: dancing, horseback riding, walking a coastal path, visiting a beautiful garden, relaxing in a sauna, or simply sitting in the hot tub. Aim to do at least one a week over the next month.

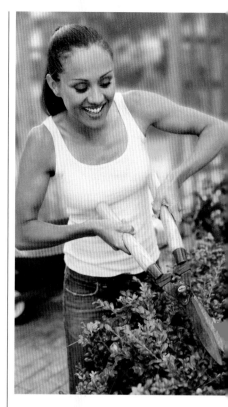

Build lifestyle-friendly exercise into your day—then you can dispense with the gym.

At least once a week treat yourself by doing something that makes you feel good.

Food is your friend

When you befriend real food, you start to recognize the nasty chemical tang of many ready-made meals for what it often is—junk. The World Health Organization (WHO) blames processed foods for the steep rise in worldwide obesity, since they often contain high levels of sugar, unhealthy fats, and salt—and tend to contain less fiber and nutrients than the raw ingredients used to make them.

Buy fresh seasonal produce, then all you need to focus on is taste.

37

Helpful flowers

The following Australian Bush Flower Essences may help if guilt or shame prevents you from enjoying the pleasure of good food. Place 4 drops in water and sip until symptoms subside.
- Billy Goat Plum: for dislike of the physical body, or self-disgust.
- Sturt Desert Pea: for guilt following over-indulgence.
- Bush Fuchsia: to listen to your intuition about what's right to eat and when.

38

Enjoy a runner's high

Engage in moderate-intensity activity for 30 minutes to stimulate a natural high; it seems to trigger the release of an amphetamine-like chemical phenylethylamine, which boosts mood and energy levels.

39

Savor wine

Sipping a glass of wine with a meal forces you to stop and savor the moment, helps to maintain healthy cholesterol levels, and reduces risk of coronary heart disease. But you don't need much to benefit—the World Health Organization recommends one drink every other day to keep the heart in shape. Drinking more can increase risk of heart and liver disease.

40

Junk the junk

Challenge yourself to eat fewer ready meals. Make one or two days a week junk food free, or avoid those aisles in your grocery store. Experiment with recipes for meals you usually enjoy ready-made—burgers, lasagna, or gumbo—and invite your household to see if they can taste the difference.

41

What's in season?

One way to ditch ready-made meals is to shop with the seasons. Focus your supermarket shopping around the fresh produce section and the fish counter, and visit www.eatwiththeseasons.com for profiles of the current season's top ingredients, from kale to sweet potatoes, as well as lots of inspiring recipes and shopping tips. Sign up for a weekly email update.

42

Taste, not nutrients

Fixating on the components of food—its nutrients or its fat, sugar, and salt content—detracts from the pleasure of eating. If you buy mostly seasonal raw ingredients—fruit, vegetables, fish—and cook them yourself, you can stop worrying about the health factor and just enjoy the flavor.

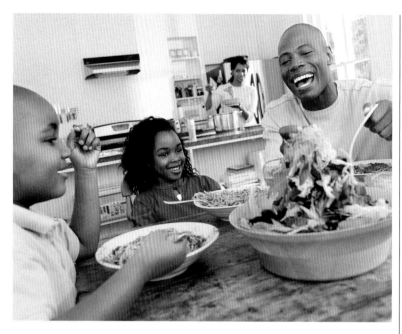

Make the most of every opportunity to enjoy traditional family mealtimes.

43
Call that food?
Food polemicist Michael Pollan argues that to eat healthily we should shun anything our great grandmothers wouldn't recognize as food—yogurt in tubes, pop tarts, breakfast bars. These products only exist because of food-processing methods that require additives, artificial colorings, and preservatives.

44
Eat like your ancestors
The World Health Organization blames the obesity epidemic both on changing patterns of eating and what we eat—eating fewer meals as a family and eating while distracted by electronic accompaniment, for example. Eat like your great grandparents during the weekend: throw a family lunch then take a siesta or a post-meal walk.

45
Guess the shape
See if you can spend a day eating only things that have a recognizable shape—tomatoes, apples, eggs, mackerel, a chicken, rice. This is an easy way to avoid processed food.

46
Enjoy real meat
If you eat meat, buy the best you can afford: try to avoid processed pies or hot dogs, but instead choose a recognizable cut from a recognizable animal—buy from a local butcher if you can. This meat tastes better and may also have health benefits. A study of almost 200,000 people carried out at the University of Hawaii found that those who ate mostly processed meat raised their risk of pancreatic cancer by 67 percent over those who rarely ate meat.

47
Follow a traditional diet
It doesn't matter whether it's Greek, Italian, Indian, or Japanese, eating the traditional foods of your cultural heritage is likely to leave you in better shape than a modern Western diet. Buy yourself a regional cookbook and master a few staples for each season.

48
Savor special occasions
Don't get so hung up on calorie counting or wholefoods that you spoil special occasions. If it's your birthday, you deserve chocolate, cake, and champagne. Just get back to your healthy eating the next day.

49
Blog about dinner
Set yourself an online challenge for the rest of the world to hold you to. Bored clerk Julie Powell, a novice cook, decided to cook all 524 dishes

in Julia Child's tome *Mastering the Art of French Cooking*, and to blog about the experience. She rediscovered her appetite for life—read about it in her book *Julie and Julia*.

50

Ditch the multivitamins

If you stop taking supplements, then you will be forced to think up new ways to get nutrients onto your plate, such as eating more fruit, vegetables, and pulses. Plant nutrients seem to work more effectively in combination with each other, with many beneficial compounds and combinations yet to be explained by science.

51

Rediscover your passion

Enjoy Thai curries? Learn how to make them by taking a class with the chef at a Thai restaurant. Love pizza? Why not splurge on a cooking class in Tuscany.

52

Simple fast food

Quality ingredients simply prepared are the secret of good eating. For a fast, hassle-free lunch, just assemble huge bowls of salad; platters of smoked fish, thin-sliced cured ham, and cheeses; loaves of artisan-baked bread; and bowls of fresh fruit.

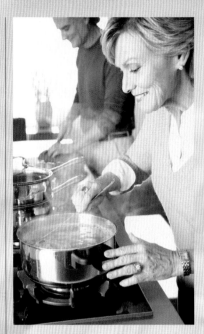

Learn new cooking skills and reignite your passion for all your favorite foods.

Keep it simple: all it takes to eat healthily is quality ingredients simply prepared.

Stay happy, stay slim

Research suggests that being overweight and feeling depressed go hand in hand, especially for women. The links go both ways: being overweight makes exercise onerous and can raise risk of depression by 20 percent, while feeling down can make you lethargic and increase your appetite. Here are some tips to help you beat the blues and stay upbeat and happy about your shape and weight.

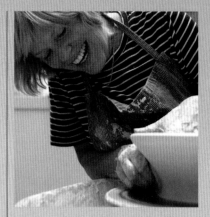

Learning a new skill is a great way to stay active and boost self-esteem.

53
Anxiety-soothing food
The amino acid tryptophan helps the brain produce the neurotransmitter serotonin, which can soothe anxiety. Tryptophan is found in healthy snacks such as dates, bananas, and mangoes; sesame, sunflower, and pumpkin seeds.

54
Chocolate on the brain
A few squares of dark chocolate can boost your mood and zest for life. Flavanols in cocoa enhance alertness, while the constituent

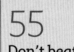

Chocolate made with at least 70 percent cocoa solids is a good mood food.

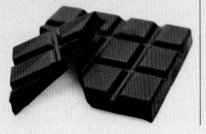

amino acid GABA reduces anxiety. Chocolate also contains tryptophan (see No. 53). But beware: this is not true of calorie-rich confectionery, which contains ingredients such as sugar and milk and sweet fillings.

55
Don't beat yourself up
People who bathe in self-criticism and negative thoughts set themselves up to fail, while positive thinking has been linked with long-term weight loss. If your first thought after missing an exercise session is "I'll never achieve my goal," acknowledge that self-criticism, then look for your second, more optimistic thought. Ask "How can I make up for it tomorrow?" or "How can I avoid that outcome next time?" A University of Pittsburgh study found that optimists tend to be less passive than pessimists; they regard setbacks as temporary and changeable, and believe their actions make a difference.

56
Worry not
The stress hormone cortisol prompts the body to lay down fat around the abdomen. So value relaxation techniques, such as massage or meditation, as important weight-loss weapons.

57
Throw a pot
Using your body to express yourself and gain a sense of achievement doesn't have to mean an intimidating exercise class. Learning to throw clay pots is a fun way to start exploring your body, especially if your weight—and others' attitudes to it – gets you down. Throwing clay on a wheel improves coordination and balance, hones upper-body strength, and encourages you to engage the core muscles in your abdomen.

59
Abdominal chanting

When you feel stressed, sit resting your palms on your lower abdomen. Take a deep breath in. As you exhale, open your mouth wide and let the sound "AAAHHH" emerge. Project it to the other side of the room and with it your stresses. As you breathe in, imagine refreshing oxygen neutralizing any tension. Repeat until you feel more upbeat.

60
Uplifting oil

Put 3–4 drops of essential oil of orange (or other favorite citrus oil) on a tissue and place on a warm radiator or directly into an oil burner in the room where you are doing uplifting yoga poses, relaxation, or chanting. The scent of citrus is uplifting for the spirits.

61
Fun flowers

The Californian Flower Essence Zinnia promotes light-heartedness and a sense of fun, which may be lacking if you have a serious outlook

58
Try juggling

Because it occupies your mind fully, when you juggle you forget your cares and don't realize you are exercising. A Japanese study found it especially good therapy for women with anxiety disorders. Practice at home, enroll in a circus skills workshop, or visit www.jugglingdb.com.

Meditation in motion: juggling releases tension and reduces anxiety while keeping you fit.

or your job involves dealing with other people's problems. Place 4 drops in water and sip until negativity subsides.

62

Smile when you're down

Pretend to be happy: studies show it makes you feel happier and more relaxed. To make yourself smile, simply think back to something that made you happy recently—maybe something amusing that a child said or a compliment at work.

63

Laughter yoga

There are more than 5,000 laughter clubs across 40 countries. As well as keeping the spirits high, laughter exercises the lungs, improves posture, and releases tension. Sample the laughter-yoga videos on YouTube.

64

Play with boys

A study of children in North Carolina showed that the longer children were overweight, the greater their risk of becoming depressed. Boys seemed particularly at risk. Make time after school to play ball or Frisbee. This boosts activity levels, self-esteem, and body image, and allows you to share in a child's infectious laughter and *joie de vivre*.

65

Blues-busting exercise

When you feel down, just 10–15 minutes of brisk exercise produces enough endorphins, the body's natural opiates, to bring on a natural high.

66

Balance the fats

Omega-6, found especially in safflower, corn, and sunflower oils (and vegetable oil blends) is essential for health. But too much blocks absorption of another vital fatty acid, omega-3. Deficiency of omega-3 may contribute to depression (and heart disease). The human body does best eating roughly equal amounts of the two, but Western diets can give us 20 or 30 times more omega-6. For balance, cut back on processed foods

Pumpkin seeds contain tryptophan and are a great source of omega-3 fatty acids.

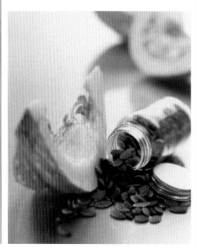

rich in vegetable oils and eat more oily fish, walnuts, pumpkin seeds, and flax (linseed) or hemp seeds or oil.

67

Happy fats

A low-fat diet can leave you feeling depressed: fat produces hormones that boost the feel-good chemical serotonin. Get yours from olive oil and oily fish—mackerel, sardines, or salmon—rather than animal fats.

68

Comfort eating

Carbohydrates are comforting to eat when you feel down—they boost production of serotonin in the brain and nervous system, helping counter depression. Choose healthy carbs such as oats, whole grains, and nuts. Sweet foods also trigger the release of opiate-like endorphins and help you to deal with pain. But make sure they are healthy sweet things, such as fresh or dried fruit.

69

Resist happy marketing

Even if the McDonald's Happy Meal has healthy options, its toy treats encourage children to favor fast-food restaurants over more "grown-up" eating places. The Happy Hour is a temptation to mainline calorie-laden drinks. It might be best to cut back on both.

Motivation matters

Motivation may be your most vital shape-up tool: unless you make real lifestyle changes and stick to them, dieting can be followed by rapid weight gain and the best-made exercise plans fall apart. Here are some ways to get from good intentions to action. Bear in mind that people who exercise regularly just get on and do it rather than thinking about it too much.

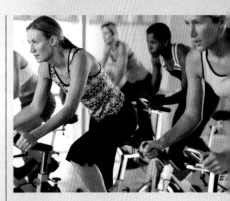

Exercising with others will help you to keep focused and motivated.

70
Plan ahead
Studies show that once you get into the habit of exercising regularly it becomes easier to keep to an exercise regime, and after only 21 sessions exercise becomes second nature. People who succeed do so because they exercise at a convenient time and place, and they factor in obstacles such as working late or rain.

71
Think of the benefits
Few people enjoy exercising at first. The ones who persevere, or for whom it becomes routine, might simply be better at talking themselves into it. Jot down a list of some of the benefits you will enjoy as a result of being in better shape and pin it or prop it up somewhere prominent: for example, beside the bathroom mirror, on the fridge, or on the back of the front door. Read through it regularly.

72
Prop up a photo
Visual people respond better to picture prompts than words. Do you have a photo of yourself in shape—maybe on holiday? Prop it up near your list of fitness benefits.

73
Enlist support
People who get fit or lose weight in groups have more staying power than those who go it alone.

Find a photo of yourself in shape and use it as a visual prompt to keep you focused on your goal.

74
Join the club
Joining a weight-loss organization can boost your motivation with its balanced diet plans, practical cooking and exercise tips, and motivational speakers, but perhaps the regular group meetings, camaraderie, and leaders who have done it themselves are more important.

75
Recruit an online buddy
Many online diet organizations (try www.realage.com) offer not only a meal and shopping planner but also a forum for meeting a diet buddy to whom you can post daily, helping you to stay on track.

76
Clarify your motivation
When motivation wanes, articulate the deep reasons underlying your wish to lose weight; this can help to keep you going. Write them down and refer back to them often.

Try the tonic herb Siberian ginseng if your energy levels for exercise are flagging.

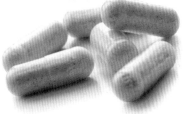

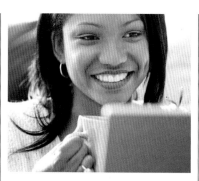

Keeping in daily contact with an online buddy may help you maintain your resolve.

77
Cancel the self-talk
Monitor your inner voice. When you hear yourself saying, "I tried that before and gave up," ask it to be quiet and instead tell yourself something positive about what you did achieve this week.

78
Think about others
List how those you love will benefit from your campaign. Will you have more energy for your partner (your sex life may well improve) and for playing with your children? And if your confidence at work gets a boost will colleagues also benefit?

79
Weight loss rewards
Research shows that rewarding good behavior is much more effective than punishing bad behavior when losing weight and keeping it off.

80
List your treats
Non-food rewards are helpful if you associate happiness with junk food. Allocate little treats for being good every day, not so little treats for keeping it up, and splurges for meeting your major targets. The first might include 10 more minutes in bed, the second a new DVD, and the last could be a weekend break or a new bag.

81
Energy tonic
If you have trouble summoning up the energy to exercise, try the tonic herb Siberian ginseng (*Eleutherococcus senticosus*), which can increase stamina and ability to cope with stress. Take in capsule or tincture form, as directed.

82
See a homeopath
If lack of energy becomes a problem, see your doctor or a homeopath. Chronic fatigue syndrome, or CFS, responds well to homeopathic treatment.

83
Just get on with it!
If you need to bust apathy and procrastination, sip the following Californian Flower Essence

combination in water (2 drops of each) until symptoms subside. It's not subtle, so use with caution!

• Blackberry: aids manifestation of ideas and decisive action.

• Cayenne: a catalyst for change.

• Tansy: cuts through lethargy and promotes action.

84

Body tune-in

After a run, a yoga session, or walking the dog, close your eyes for 30 seconds and notice how you feel. Happy, elated, calm? When willpower wavers, close your eyes and recall those motivational sensations.

85

Change your family

Enlist your family's support for your lifestyle changes. Plan fun activities together such as regular swim or rollerblading sessions.

86

Professional support

Can you enlist professional help—personal trainer, nutritionist, counselor—to keep you motivated?

87

Find a spiritual mentor

Aro gTér Buddist organization runs a down-to-earth meditation mentoring program on its website (www.arobuddhism.org) as well as a free meditation course with weekly emails focusing on combatting boredom, frustration, and procrastination.

88

Try warrior pose

For warrior-determination, stand with your feet hip-width apart and breathe deeply. On your next inhalation, step your feet wide apart and stretch out your arms at shoulder height. Turn your left foot in a little and your right leg and foot out by 90 degrees. Exhale, stare in a determined way along your right arm, and bend your right knee toward a right angle. Take up to five breaths, then come up and repeat to the left.

Plan fun activities with your family to include them in your new lifestyle.

Master your cravings

It's all too easy to lapse from a more healthy way of living. For example, a 1996 study of would-be non-smokers found that 70 percent of those who admitted to occasional lapses had relapsed fully within three months. Here are some ways to counter the desire for the forbidden.

89
Don't lose control

If you lose control of your cravings and end up eating a whole tub of ice cream, it's then tempting to let go completely and open a package of cookies, too, with the thought that your healthy diet resumes tomorrow. But be aware that the mind scrambles to take advantage of breaks in restrictions, and think twice before giving in to temptation.

Detach yourself from cravings using mind-screen meditation.

90
Love your future

Don't see a relapse as proof of weakness and project it into future actions. This is thinking like an addict. If you believe the cause of the failure is within you, you give yourself the freedom to relapse again. Be confident that you have the ability to change; this enhances the likelihood of success.

91
Meditate

At times of crisis, meditation builds calmness—it switches on the parasympathetic nervous system, which dampens down the body's stress responses and encourages you to look at your behavior honestly, without anger or guilt.

92
Mind-screen meditation

Close your eyes and imagine a screen behind them on which your thoughts are projected. Watch your cravings and guilt for a while as if watching a movie. Now detach yourself from them. They are still there, but don't allow your mind to follow them. They are not you. Think for a while about what you are if you are not those thoughts and feelings. Try to contact this deep, still "you" within.

93
Rediscover your faith

Studies show that going to a house of worship influences lifestyle habits in a positive way, including keeping non-smokers on the straight and narrow. Can you explore your own faith tradition to find ways to deepen your spiritual life? In studies, it is the regularity of attendance at places of worship and the community support that seems especially nurturing.

94
Prayer for serenity

The prayer adopted by Alcoholics Anonymous helps those facing daily issues: "God grant me the serenity to accept the things I cannot change, courage to change the things I can, and wisdom to know the difference."

95
Yoga resolve

Seek out a teacher (or DVD) of Satyananda Yoga Nidra, a type of yoga formulated to overcome distractions of the mind, and learn how to set yourself a *sankalpa* or positive statement of resolve.

96
Relaxation yoga

Sitting cross-legged, work through this sequence with patience. If you can't reach the floor in the first step, place a chair in front of you and stretch forward on to the seat. **Stretch forward** over your right knee, keeping your left knee down and buttocks on the floor. Repeat over your left knee, then to the front. **Lie back** and stretch your arms over your head or to the sides. Breathe softly. Sit up, change the cross of your legs, and repeat the stretch. **To finish**, still lying on your back, uncross your legs, pull your knees into your chest and rock them back and forth to massage your lower back.

97
Calming herbs

To reduce anxiety while giving up smoking (or anything else you use as an emotional crutch), let a combination of the herbs *Avena*

98
Squat it off

Try this hard-hitting exercise to get your mind off of temptation and on to your aching (toning) bottom and thighs. Work up to three sets of 5–10 reps of each of these three squats.

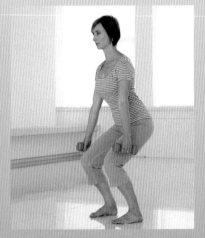

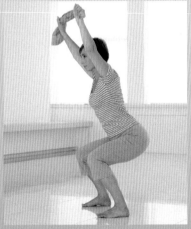

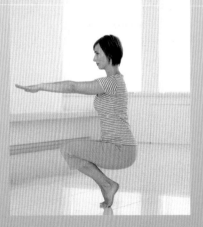

1 Stand with feet hip-width apart holding light weights. Bend your knees to lower yourself, back straight. Push through your heels to stand up.

2 Repeat with arms raised overhead, holding a scarf to keep your arms straight. Look forward and keep your knees over your little toes.

3 Stand with feet together on tip-toes, arms outstretched. Sink into a squat, heels raised. Try to lift back to your starting position on tiptoes.

sativa, *Scutellaria*, and *Valerian* support your nervous system and help you stay on an even keel. Put 5 drops of each tincture in a glass of water and drink twice a day.

99
Sugar remedies

If you have a sweet tooth, the Australian Bush Flower Essence Peach Flowered Tea Tree may help. It reduces sugar cravings and mood swings caused by yo-yoing blood sugar. Take with the essence Wedding Bush to support your commitment to an exercise or diet regime. Place 4 drops in water and sip until symptoms subside.

100
Mood food

In smoking studies, being in a bad mood was the second most common trigger for relapse (behind smoking cues such as drinking or socializing); some studies increased cravings by inducing negativity in volunteers. Try some of the good-mood strategies on pages 18–20.

101
Get more magnesium

Magnesium deficiency may contribute to cravings for chocolate or cookies before a woman's menstrual period. Get more magnesium into your diet by eating pumpkin seeds, nuts, almonds, and cashews, and eat spinach and white fish, such as halibut.

102
Just 10 minutes

To stave off cravings, do 10 minutes of activity that leaves you slightly breathless. Perhaps walk up and down stairs when others have a cigarette break. That counts as a workout, and people who do one are likely to do more.

103
Peak activity

Cravings tend to peak in late afternoon or early evening. Be prepared by keeping some coping strategies and distractions close at hand to minimize the risk of a full-blown relapse.

104
Pre-planned distractions

Distractions work best if they're slightly naughty: an erotic novel, gossip website, sexy texting, or a brisk stroll to the shoe store.

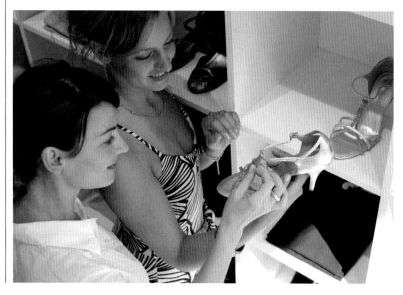

Distract yourself from your cravings by doing something a little extravagant!

105
Get home delivery
If you crack at the supermarket, stop going in person and book a delivery instead. Make a master list of healthy staple foods on a supermarket shopping site and just press deliver each week. No pester power, no temptation, no guilt: just healthy food delivered directly to your door.

106
Brush your teeth
After a meal, brush your teeth; when your teeth feel squeaky-clean, you are less likely to snack or pick at leftovers. This also works if you're trying to limit yourself to one or two glasses of wine.

107
Text a friend
When you relapse, confide what happened to a sympathetic friend. Next time you're tempted, text her for support. In one study into stopping smoking, this proved to be a successful aid.

108
Cognitive approaches
In smoking studies, lapses weren't prevented by behavioral strategies such as drinking water or deep breathing, but by changing thought patterns. To do this, think of yourself as an active person, revisit the reasons you want to live more healthily, act positive, and focus on distracting your mind.

109
Thought-distraction exercise
Buy two pairs of silly glasses, each a different color. Name one pair the cravings glasses. Put them on when you're tempted and let your mind wallow in why you want to watch TV rather than go to the gym or why that chocolate bar is so desirable. Now put on the other pair—your healthy glasses. Look at your cravings from their viewpoint: can you understand how good you'll feel after class, and how bad you'll feel after eating that chocolate bar?

110
Brainstorm challenges
List the challenges standing in the way of your goals: I snack when I have a glass of wine; I work too late to get to the gym; I have no childcare. Brainstorm solutions to each one, perhaps as a mind map. So, if lack of childcare is stopping you from exercising you might find a mother and toddler gym session or plan to go for a brisk walk in the park with your baby in the stroller.

111
Quality over quantity
Look for high-quality versions of favorite treats: very good-quality dark chocolate, jewel-like pâtisserie pastries, and artisan cider. Generally, you'll require less to feel satisfied.

High-quality treats will satisfy you quicker so you need to eat less of them.

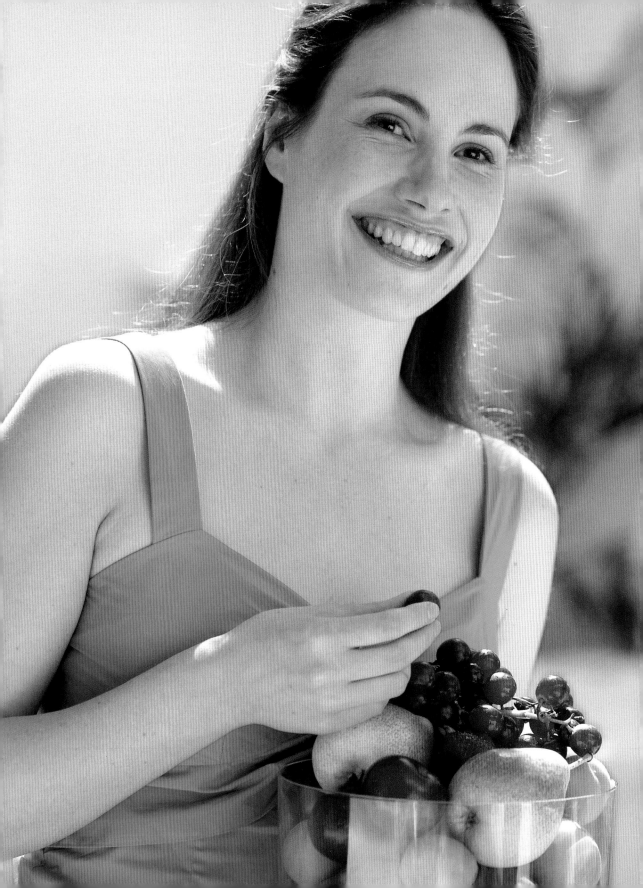

2 Healthy at home

Time has become a scarce resource—there are just not enough hours in the day to work, shop, cook, and go to the gym or get active with the kids. In the US we work much longer hours than our European counterparts, and have fewer days off, both of which are major causes of high stress levels. Working long hours also correlates with increased exhaustion and depression, leaving mind as well as body out of shape. When we spend this long working, it pays dividends to make the home a haven of fitness-friendly foods and activities to stop us dropping, exhausted, onto the sofa with a large glass of wine and a TV dinner. This chapter shows easy ways to do so, from filling a fruit bowl to making use of the green gym just outside the back door.

Wake up well

Each new day brings an opportunity to start afresh, and if you're a busy person, then first thing in the morning can be the best time for a gentle yoga session or a walk with the dog. Later in the day other tasks will often seem more urgent. A Glasgow University study found that people who exercised in the morning enhanced their mood by 30 percent, which is significantly more than those who exercised in the evening.

112
Set the alarm
Waking up at the same time each day—weekends included – makes us feel more refreshed and alert, say sleep experts. They believe that getting into a consistent daily waking routine regularizes our circadian rhythms, the internal body clock that determines our waking, sleeping, and eating patterns.

Harness your body's natural energy by rising with the sun.

113
Rise with the sun
Waking before the sun rises increases energy, teach practitioners of India's ancient system of healthcare, Ayurveda. It harnesses *vata*, the energy of movement and fresh activity, which is at its peak from around 2am until dawn.

114
Dawn light
If you live away from streetlights, sleep with the curtains open to encourage awakening with the light of dawn. Some people, especially those with seasonal affective disorder, feel more alert and less depressed when they use dawn-simulation lamp alarms, which simulate a slow sunrise.

115
Gain morning minutes
In order to gain more minutes for exercise in the morning, every third day set your alarm clock 15 minutes earlier. Before two weeks is out, you will have gained an extra hour in your day. Use this time to do some gentle, awakening exercise and start your day on a high.

116

Drink water

After a night's sleep, your body may be dehydrated. Drink a large glass of fresh water on waking to kickstart your digestive and excretory systems.

117

Morning thought

While other household members doze, spend 10–20 minutes preparing your mind for an active day. Sit with legs crossed and spine straight. Rest the backs of your hands on your knees. Close your eyes and feel your breath moving in and out, noticing the refreshingly cool air on your nostrils on the inhalation. As you breathe in, silently repeat your intention for the day: "I am vital and alert" or "I will meet every obstacle with energy."

118

Wake your feet

Before morning exercise, warm your feet with a quick self-massage using your favorite invigoratingly scented body lotion or foot cream.

Cross one foot onto your opposite knee and massage all over with lotion. Using long, soothing strokes with both palms, work around the sole and toes, over the top of the foot, around the ankle, and into the Achilles tendon in the lower calf.

Holding the top of the foot in your fingers, press both thumbs into the sole, making tiny circles down the sides, from the heel to the base of the toes. Repeat to cover the sole. **Massage each toe** in turn between fingers and thumb, stretching out the toe and pressing at the tip. Finish by circling the foot from the ankle in one direction then the other. Repeat on your other foot.

119

Yoga mat spritzer

Infusing your mat with an energizing aroma can help you stick to an early morning routine. Cedarwood aids meditation and motivation, rosemary clears the head and dissolves lethargy, and geranium lifts the spirits. Use fresh oils only.

2 tsp grapeseed oil
3 drops each essential oils of
  cedarwood, rosemary, and geranium

Spoon the grapeseed oil into a bottle with a spritzer pump, then drop in the essential oils. Add 3 tablespoons of water. Screw on the top and shake. Spritz the air around your mat before an exercise session. Keep the bottle in the fridge for up to a week.

120

Yoga for digestion

Sit cross-legged with your hands palm down on your knees. Lengthen the back of your neck and spine and draw your chin in. Exhale fully and

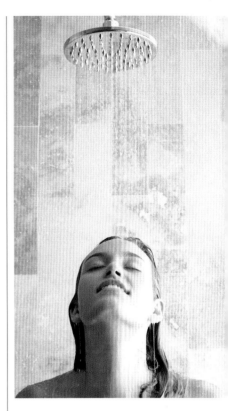

Enhance the invigorating effects of your shower with a peppermint shower gel.

then, holding your breath, suck your abdomen up and draw your belly button toward your spine. Relax and inhale. Repeat twice more. (Avoid if you have any medical condition other than minor digestive problems.)

121

Peppermint shower gel

For extra invigoration, stir 2 drops of essential oil of peppermint into 2 tablespoons of unscented shower gel just before showering. (Avoid if you are pregnant, breastfeeding, or have sensitive skin.)

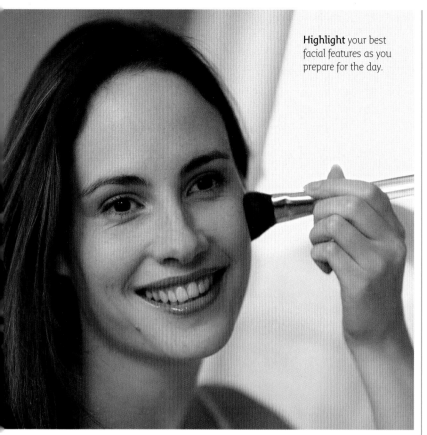

Highlight your best facial features as you prepare for the day.

in artery-clogging fat). Persevere even if your gums bleed; after a few days they will be more robust.

125
Face-shaping make-up tricks

Emphasizing your best features guides the eye from areas you'd rather forget about. When getting ready for the day, highlight great cheekbones with a brush of light-reflecting powder, make up beautiful eyes, or paint lips a striking color to draw attention down the face.

126
Facial exercise sequence

Many women swear that exercising the facial muscles keeps the face in shape through the decades. These morning exercises are for the eyes.
Keeping your head still, look up with your eyes and hold. Then look down; don't lower your chin. Look as far to the left as you can, then right. Look to the top left and bottom right; top right and bottom left. Circle your eyes around an imaginary clock-face. Repeat counterclockwise.
Widen your eyes as much as possible and hold. Don't lift your eyebrows. Keeping your eyes wide, open your mouth as far as you can and stick out your tongue. Can you touch your chin?
Close your eyes, scrunch up your face, and hold. Repeat step 2.

122
Rosemary bath

To lift morning fatigue, the Ayurvedic tradition recommends a rosemary bath. Pick a handful of fresh sprigs, secure with a rubber band, and throw under the hot tap while the bath fills.

123
Bathroom rave

To boost circulation, put on some up-tempo music and dance as you dry. Punch to the ceiling, circle your shoulders, flap your arms like a chicken, lift alternate knees to meet opposite hands, pummel your chest Tarzan-like, and shake out your limbs, hands, and feet.

124
Clean teeth, clean arteries

After cleaning your teeth, work floss gently between the top of your teeth and gums to keep your gums and heart in shape. Studies show that people with gum disease have a higher risk of heart disease (the bacteria in plaque has been found

A hearty breakfast

An American study found that people who ate breakfast had a higher daily intake of vitamins, minerals, and whole grains. People who regularly skip breakfast tend to weigh more, and in some studies eating breakfast seems to correlate with significant long-term weight loss. However, not all breakfasts are alike ...

127
The night before
Set the breakfast table before you go to bed and save precious minutes in the morning. To tempt non-breakfast eaters, you can also set the bread machine so that it starts making bread in the early hours. Not only will this fill the house with an irresistible aroma, but you will also have delicious, healthy homemade bread for breakfast.

128
For delicate stomachs
If you can't face breakfast, drink a cup of camomile tea 30 minutes before eating. It soothes digestion and prevents nausea.

129
Improve your appetite
Aloe vera stimulates bile flow, aiding digestion. If you suffer from habitual constipation or lack appetite in the mornings, take this herb in tincture or capsule form according to pack instructions.

130
Make mine fiber
People who eat the fiber found in whole grains tend to have a lower risk of cardiovascular disease and type 2 diabetes. Some studies suggest it slows weight gain and keeps your BMI (see No. 8) healthy, too. Check the label and favor cereals with 4g fiber per portion.

131
Check your portion
Pour your regular cereal in your regular bowl and weigh it. How does that relate to the suggested portion (and calorie count) on the box? Now weigh out the recommended portion and pour into the bowl. Do you need a smaller bowl?

132
Oat so healthy
Eating whole oats reduces the risk of coronary heart disease. It may also lower cholesterol and help improve blood pressure, treat type 2 diabetes, and maintain a healthy weight. A simple way to eat oats is in oatmeal.

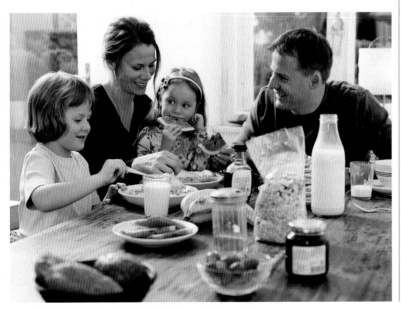

Get your family's day off to the best start possible with a nutritious breakfast.

133
Fruit oatmeal

This is low in fat and sugar; it's also delicious and filling (feeling full at breakfast results in fewer calories being taken in during the day). The apricots and banana make it sweet enough not to require sugar. Serves 4.

1 cup jumbo organic oats
2½ cups skim or semi-skim milk
handful apricots, chopped
1 banana, thinly sliced
8 cardamom pods

Place the oats and milk in a large pan over low heat. Stir in the fruit. Crush the cardamom pods with a pestle or the handle of a heavy knife, then throw into the pan. Slowly bring to a boil, stirring constantly. Take off the heat and leave for 5 minutes to allow the oats to plump up before serving. Drizzle with maple syrup for a delicious treat.

134
Pour a pint

To keep your bones (and blood pressure) in shape, you need about 2½ cups of milk daily (or two cups of yogurt or 3oz/80g hard cheese). Calcium builds bone mass up to the age of 30–35, then maintains it, to keep you exercising safely into older age. If you dislike milk on cereal, fix yourself a latte, a bowl of plain yogurt, or top a whole grain bagel with grated cheese.

135
Froth it up

Low-fat and skim milk contain all the calcium of full fat or whole milk, but much less fat. To make skim milk

Boost bone density with a glass of milk a day. You can build much of this quota into breakfast.

more palatable in coffee, warm it to boiling point, then whizz with a cappuccino frother.

136
Refresh your coffee
Adopt an Eastern Mediterranean tradition and drink a glass of water with your morning coffee; this leaves you feeling both fuller and better hydrated.

137
Two or more
The US government recommends that we eat 9–13 portions of fruit and vegetables daily. It's easy to build at least two of these into breakfast. Pour a glass of pure fruit juice and chop pieces of fresh fruit over cereal. Try to choose seasonal or different colored fruit.

138
Soak some fruit
Before bed, place a handful of prunes in a bowl and cover with water. By morning you have a plump and tasty addition to muesli that is high in fiber and potassium.

139
Eat whole fruit
Whole fruit is healthiest because it contains fiber, which can be lost in pressing when making fruit juice.

140
Cloudy juices
Choose cloudy, or non-clarified, apple juice. Polish researchers found it contains up to four times more polyphenols. These antioxidants keep us in shape by mopping up cell-damaging free radicals, offering protection from heart disease and cancer.

141
Potassium shake
Eating a potassium-rich diet helps maintain healthy blood pressure. However, the 2005 US Dietary Guidelines Advisory Committee found that no age group surveyed consumed the recommended amount. This smoothie contains fruit high in potassium.

handful of dried apricots
large slice cantaloupe or honeydew melon, seeded
freshly squeezed juice of 1 orange
3 tbsp plain yogurt

Place all the ingredients in a blender and process until well combined. Pour into a glass.

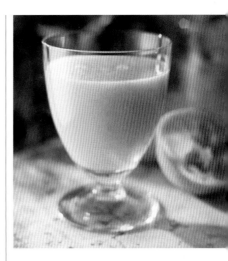

A glass of pure fruit juice will start you off on your recommended five (or more) a day.

142
Start a breakfast club
Start a breakfast club for kids on the weekends or the morning after sleepovers, encouraging them to cook eggs, pancakes or waffles with you.

143
Copycats
A Finnish study found that adolescents tend to eat like their parents. To be a better role model, place fruit salad and a carton of quality smoothie on the table or serve up eggs. Make this a time when you sit and eat with your children.

Potassium rich: fruits such as cantaloupe are high in this essential nutrient.

Housework workout

The key to becoming more active is not to think of exercise as something you go to a special place to do—the gym, the pool, or at a yoga studio, for example—but as something that feels as natural as climbing the stairs. There are plenty of opportunities around the home to make your day more active. Finding tasks that add up to 30 minutes a day most days of the week isn't difficult if you follow these tips.

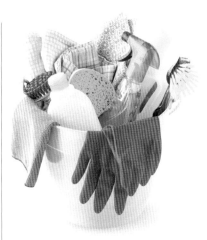

144
Stay active

A Dutch study in the journal *Nature* found that people who engaged in moderate-intensity activity were more active overall than those who occasionally upped the intensity of their activity. We need to burn 400 calories a day in physical activity to stay in shape: 30 minutes of vacuuming burns 105, and walking briskly up and down stairs putting toys and clothes away without stopping burns up to 150.

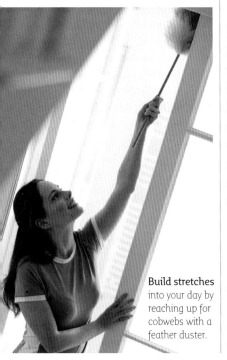

Build stretches into your day by reaching up for cobwebs with a feather duster.

145
Balance board warm up

Keep a "wobble" board at home and use it to awaken your senses and body awareness before starting a housework session. This also builds core strength and a flexible pelvis and trunk. Spherical boards that move through 360 degrees are more effective than rockers that move from side to side.

146
Ditch the appliances

To sustain moderate activity, wash and dry dishes by hand instead of using a dishwater, use a dustpan and brush over a vacuum cleaner, walk the clothes to the backyard to hang them out to dry rather than going straight to the dry cycle. All this makes your home greener, too.

Back to basics: put on your rubber gloves and get to grips with some manual cleaning.

147
Dusting stretches

Buy a feather duster and practice this stretch as you swipe at cobwebs. **Holding the duster** in your right hand, stand with feet hip-width apart and stretch it toward the ceiling. Lengthen your right side from hip to underarm without letting your left side collapse. **Still stretching up,** inhale. As you exhale, pull your tummy muscles in and reach over your head to your left side. Keep the left side of your waist long and stop if you feel strain on your back. **Come back to the center** and repeat the sideways stretch 5 times. Repeat on your left side.

Get onto your hands and knees to scrub the kitchen floor—this works your back and abdominal muscles.

148

Floor scrubbing

Being on your hands and knees is a good position to get into if your life is sedentary. It stretches your upper back and activates the core muscles in your abdomen, which support your frame.

Get onto hands and knees, hands under your shoulders and knees beneath your hips. Circle your hips clockwise, then counterclockwise. Then lengthen your spine from tailbone to the crown of your head, making a tabletop shape.

Press on your hands and push the top of your back toward the ceiling, making an "n" shape. Relax your head and neck.

Holding the position, exhale, pulling your abdominal muscles back and up. Inhale and return to the tabletop position. Repeat a few times. Now scrub the floor, making wide circles clockwise and counterclockwise, using both hands.

149

Clean to the beat

Put on some high-energy music when tidying or cleaning, and coordinate your movements with the beat. Or spend the first five minutes dancing around to warm up before getting down to work. Have another five-minute dance once you have finished, making your movements slower and smaller as you cool down.

150

Squat pick-up

Picking up toys or laundry from the floor is a great excuse to work your thighs and buttocks. Stand with feet hip-width apart with the objects within arm's reach. Inhale; and as you exhale pull in your tummy muscles, then bend at the knees and hips, squatting low enough to pick the item up easily. Inhale as you come back to standing. Squat for each item. If your children scatter the floor with toys daily, you'll notice a difference in your shape in a couple of weeks.

151

Start a family chore list

To get the whole household active, draw up a chore list that assigns tasks. Make sure everyone gets a good mix of duties: carrying heavy garbage cans, scrubbing the bathtub, raking the yard, washing windows, and mowing the lawn count as high intensity; washing the dishes,

putting away dishes, and setting the table count as moderate.

152

Be mindful

Practitioners of Eastern exercise systems, such as t'ai chi or yoga, teach that the energy that fires us up emanates from the *hara*, a well of energy sited around the navel. As you do housework, imagine each movement starting in this core part of the body and radiating out to your extremities, and visualize your breath fanning a flame of motivating energy here.

153

Wear massage sandals

Take a cool-down stroll wearing massage sandals after a housework session; allow the tiny fingers on the footbed to massage away aches and to promote circulation—this will help oxygenate your cells and carry away toxins. Reflexologists teach that as you stimulate points on the soles of the feet, you enhance the well-being of other parts of the body. The heels—where you land before transferring your weight forward—relate to the pelvis, buttocks, and sciatic nerve.

154

Arm workout

If you have loose rugs, clean them the old-fashioned way with a carpet beater or big stick. This exercises first your chest muscles and the biceps, then the muscles in your shoulders and the triceps at the back of your arms.

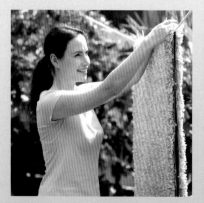

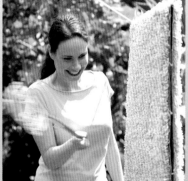

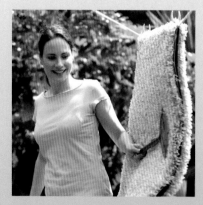

1 Throw the rug over a clothesline, the higher the line, the better. For extra security as you beat, attach clothespins to keep it in place.

2 Standing sideways, with your left shoulder next to the rug and holding the beater in your right hand, swing your shoulders to beat the rug.

3 After two minutes, change direction and beat "backhand." Move to the back of the rug, place the beater in your left hand, and repeat.

Reshape your home

You can boost the amount of activity in your day by rethinking the way you use your home. A US study found that a quarter of Americans did no physical activity in their leisure time, but we need 30 minutes most days to stay healthy, 60 minutes to prevent weight gain, and 90 minutes to sustain weight loss. The most profound change you can make is to move the TV.

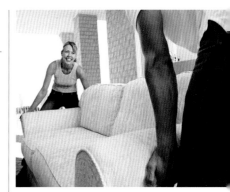

Does your sofa offer support? If yours is soft, swap it for one that supports your back.

155
Move the TV
If the TV dominates your living space, you're more likely to flip it on just out of habit. Can you move it somewhere less easy to reach, or adjust your seating arrangements? Why not move your most comfortable chair to a window to encourage activities such as painting or sewing?

156
Ditch some TVs
The average US viewer watches over four hours of television a day—a figure that is predicted to rise. The typical US home has more TVs (2.73) than people (2.55) found Nielsen Media Research—and the UK is catching up as flat screen technology makes it easier than ever to fit them in. According to this study, only 19 percent of homes own just one TV, but that's the way to go if you want to stay active. Consider ditching that extra TV!

157
Radio active
Try swapping TV for radio, then you can keep gardening, cleaning, or cooking as you listen. Use the hourly news bulletin as a reminder to do something active—perhaps climb the stairs while you listen. Wind-up radios burn extra calories.

158
Time shift your viewing
Record TV programs you really want to watch, then view them just before bedtime, leaving early evening free for activity and preventing mindless channel-flipping. It also stops mindless eating: one study of students found the more they watched, the more they ate.

159
Have a media-free day
A Ball State University study found that the typical American spends more time using media technology— TV, Internet, phones, video games, iPod—than any other daily activity. About nine hours a day! To make time for more activity, institute a technology ban a couple of nights a week or one weekend day. To stop temptation, lock the handsets away!

160
Beware of comfy chairs
The longer you spend sitting, the more you stress your spine and limit your range of movement. Experts recommend moving after 50 minutes. Write a reminder on a sticky note and stick it to the TV.

161
Change that chair
A soft sofa is not good for posture: look for one that feels supportive and has adequate lower-back support—the back of the sofa should support your back when your feet are flat on the floor.

DIY calorie burn: painting and decorating uses almost 150 calories per 30 minutes.

164
Do some DIY
Painting and decorating burns almost 150 calories per 30 minutes and is good exercise for the hands and forearms. Turn off the TV a couple of evenings a week in the summer (when light lasts longer) to work on your home. Stretch out your arms afterwards to avoid soreness the next day.

162
Firm chair leg stretch
Sit with feet flat on the floor and your back and head supported by the sofa back. Place your knees hip-width apart and rest your palms on your thighs. Exhaling, extend your right leg, keeping your knees in line, foot flexed. Hold as you inhale, then point your toe as you exhale. Inhale and flex your foot; exhale and lower to the floor. Repeat on the left. Repeat up to 5 times.

163
Sit on the floor
Encourage children to squat on the floor to play. Sitting in chairs shortens the hip flexor and hamstring muscles, which can lead to back problems. For watching TV, have them kneel for 10–20 minutes with knees together and buttocks either on the heels or on the floor between their legs.

165
Post-DIY arm rotation
Stand with your arms by your sides, make fists, and start to circle your hands firmly in one direction. Inhaling, take your arms up overhead, continuing to rotate from the wrist. At the top, exhale, and rotate your fists in the other direction as you slowly bring your arms down. Repeat.

166
Make long-term plans
Break down large DIY projects into bite-sized chunks to keep you active over several weekends and avoid injury or repetitive strain if you are sedentary during the week. Build a mix of activities into any one day, from sanding to painting to hanging wallpaper: spending more than two hours on the same task carries the risk of damaging ligaments and tendons.

167
Supersize your fruit bowl

Make a large fruit bowl the focus of your living room or kitchen – it can look as attractive as a flower display.

168
Raise some plants

Houseplants such as the spider plant, peace lily, and bamboo palm filter harmful airborne pollutants given off by paint, cleaning products, and tobacco smoke, helping to keep the lungs in good shape. They also seem to boost immunity: in one survey, people who lived in residential homes with lots of greenery were less prone to infections.

169
Freecycle a dining table

How can you sit down to a family meal if you have no table? Log on to the recycling site www.freecycle.org to find someone in your area giving away a table—and chairs—for free.

170
Buy new plates

Research shows that the more food there is on your plate, the more you eat, no matter how hungry you are. Search out medium-sized dinner plates, and smaller bowls and mugs than you currently use.

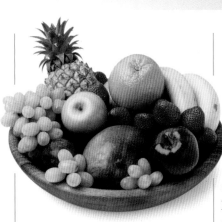

A large bowl of fruit will invite healthy eating while also looking attractive.

171
Hang mirrors

Don't reserve mirrors for the bathroom: place one where you get dressed, one where you exercise, and another where you eat. In one study, people who ate in front of a mirror reduced their food intake by almost a third.

172
Make a yoga zone

Clearing a permanent space in your home for yoga or t'ai chi motivates you to practice between classes. If space is tight, look for anywhere that allows room for you to stretch your arms overhead and to the side, perhaps next to your bed or bath or even in a garden shed. Stack everything you need close by: yoga blocks, a blanket, bolsters. For inspiration, add motivating photos or paintings, flowers, candles, or incense.

173
Park one street away

Don't curse if someone nabs the parking spot outside your front door—instead, see it as an opportunity to add activity to your day, especially if you are armed with bags full of shopping. Make a point of regularly choosing to park one or two streets away and enjoy the exercise as you stroll to and from your house.

174
Build a woodpile

Chopping wood burns as many calories per hour as basketball or aerobics. If you have an open fire or wood burner, make your next order of logs unsplit, or stop buying kindling and make it yourself.

Get active in the winter months by chopping your own logs and kindling.

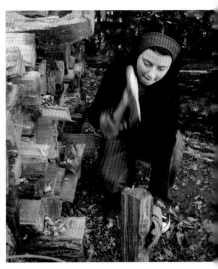

Your home gym

Gyms can be intimidating for novices and mind-numbing for regulars. So avoid them. You have all you need at home for an effective training regime—including cardiovascular, strength-building, and weight-bearing activities—from improvised weights (your baby in a sling) to a running track (around the block). Aim for at least 30 minutes of moderate-intensity activity most days, plus 6–8 strength-training exercises two days a week.

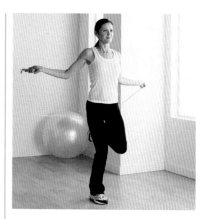

Jumping rope provides one of the best cardio workouts—find space to skip at home.

175
Mood music

Make a motivating mixed CD to encourage exercise sessions. Start with slower tracks, then build up to high-energy music before slowing down again. You control the sounds in your home gym, so tailor them precisely to your preferences rather than putting up with the tiresome techno you might find at the gym; whether you love chamber music or tango, you'll find music to inspire and raise your heart rate.

176
Jump rope

A jump rope is the ideal piece of equipment for your home gym—it is easy to store and inexpensive, and provides one of the best cardio workouts there is, toning the upper arms and legs as well as the heart and lungs. Choose a professional speed rope—the lightweight type used in skipping competitions. To check that the length is generous enough for your height, when you stand on the center of the cord, the handles should reach to your underarms.

177
Digital ropes

Digital jump ropes count the time you spend jumping and the number of reps: some allow you to input your weight and track your calorie loss. For weight training, check out ropes with removable weights in the handles.

178
Skipping steps

Skip rope for three minutes with a one-minute breather between rounds. Experiment with turning the rope forward and backward, landing on both or alternate feet or with feet together or apart, jogging with high knees or with the tops of your feet kicking your buttocks.

179
Household weights

The following are easily available, but if you prefer targeted weight-training exercises, it's safest to buy a set of home weights:
- Cans of soup
- Large milk bottle with handle (full)
- Backpack filled with groceries
- Bags of compost
- Full watering can
- Baby in a sling

180
Bicep curls

Hold weights in each hand (begin with light weights, increasing weight as you get stronger), and think about maintaining good posture throughout.
Stand with feet hip-width apart, hips over ankles, and shoulders over hips. Draw your chin in slightly. Rest your arms by your sides.

Pull your tummy muscles toward your lower back. Exhaling, tuck your elbows into your waist and raise your hands, palms facing up, to your shoulders. Exhale and lower your arms.

Repeat up to 15 times, keeping the movements flowing and in time with your breath. Do not jerk or move other parts of your body. Build up to 3 sets.

181

Use a mirror

Practice exercises with weights in front of a mirror to check your alignment and posture. Common problems include allowing your back muscles to do the work of the arms or legs, stooping, standing with one hip higher than the other, or with your feet facing in different directions.

182

How to hula

Choose an adult-sized hoop from sports stores or websites, especially if you're a beginner (they rotate more slowly and are easier to keep in the air). Use it as a three-minute cardio workout in a circuit, as a warm-up before strength training, or as a screen break if you work from home.

Have fun hula hooping your way to fitness: encourage your family to join in.

Stand with one foot in front of the other. Place the back of the hoop against your back, between your waist and chest.

Spin the hoop and move your torso forward and back—not side-to-side or in a circle which makes the hoop drop.

Persevere! Try spinning the hoop clockwise and counterclockwise.

183
Dolphin Pose

Kneel on all fours, then rest your elbows and lower arms on the floor. Clasp your hands together to make a firm triangular shape. Keeping your elbows on the floor, inhale and lift your bottom to the ceiling. Lift your body weight back and look forward. As you exhale, move your body forward and see if you can touch your chin to your thumbs without collapsing. Inhale and push back again. Repeat until you feel tired.

184
Simple circuit

Circuit training alternates cardiovascular activities with resistance training, and is easy to do at home. Set up five activities: steps to climb, bicep curls with weights, squatting holding weights, jumping rope, and crunches. Spend three minutes on each activity, moving directly from one to the other. This gives a 15-minute workout. Work up to three repetitions (45 minutes in total) three times a week.

185
Pole dancing kit

A pole dancing kit comes with a removable pole that screws into the ceiling and a DVD to show you all the moves. It's great for cardio fitness and upper body strength.

186

Yoga arm toning

This sequence takes you from the Downward Dog Pose (step 1) to the Plank Pose (step 2) and back, using only body weight to give the arm and chest muscles an effective workout.

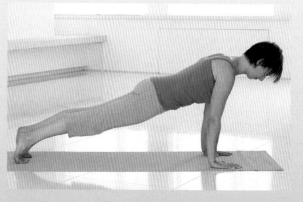

1 Kneel on all fours. Inhale and lift your bottom to the ceiling by straightening your legs and pushing back from your palms. As you exhale, push your weight toward your heels. Relax your head and neck and hold the pose.

2 Inhaling, keep your arms and legs straight and hinge forward to bring your body parallel to the floor, shoulders over wrists. Hold, then push back into Downward Dog. Switch between the two poses.

187

Convert a space

If you have the luxury of space and budget, why not convert part of a basement, garage, or garden shed into a home gym? Don't forget to check building regulations (consider insulation and ventilation) and whether the floor can take the weight of exercise machinery. The essentials are cardiovascular strengthening equipment (an exercise bike, treadmill, or rowing machine) and either a set of weights and a bench or, for those with more space and funds, a multi-gym.

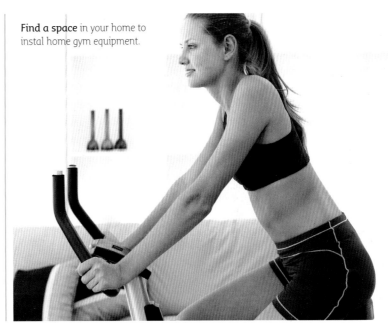

Find a space in your home to instal home gym equipment.

188

Crunches

Do one minute of crunches between three minutes of jumping rope—a boxer's warm-up. You'll need a chair with a firm seat. Repeat both lifts up to 15 times and on each side, building up to three sets.

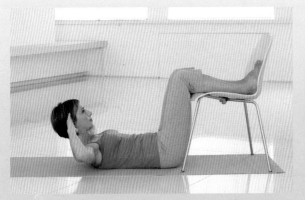

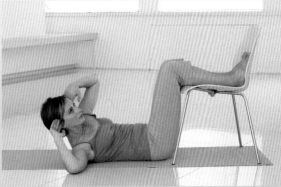

1 Lie on your back resting your calves on the seat. Shift so your knees are over your hips. Cup your hands behind your ears. Exhaling, squeeze your abdomen and raise your head and shoulders. Breathe in and lower yourself.

2 Now repeat the lift, guiding your right elbow toward your left knee as you come up. Repeat to the opposite side. Before you lift, draw your tummy toward your spine. If your tummy bulges, you have come up too high.

The lean pantry

Clearing out kitchen cupboards removes sources of temptation and stimulates a burst of motivating energy. Aim to do it twice a year, exercising your arm muscles with some scrubbing before you refill them with appetizing healthy ingredients. You might refresh the insides of cupboards with a touch of paint. Use a light, bright color—blue is thought to be appetite-suppressing.

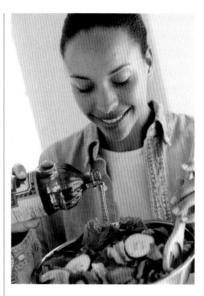

Get some of the fat your body needs from healthy oils such as olive and avocado.

189
Throw out the wrong fats

Cut down on saturated fats, which increase your risk of elevated LDL (bad) cholesterol in your blood. They come mainly from animals: most are found in full-fat cheese, milk, and in beef, with lesser amounts in ice cream, cookies, and yogurt.

190
Which bottle of oil?

We need fats every day for energy, to absorb vitamins, and repair the body. They also make food taste good. The best tasting don't leave you feeling deprived. These are olive, walnut, avocado, and hemp oil. Get the rest of your oils from oily fish to keep your brain and heart in shape.

191
How much fish?

Oily fish (and some shellfish) contain omega-3 fatty acids that keep the heart and brain healthy, so fill your cupboards with canned sardines, herring, mackerel, and anchovies, and your fridge with salmon, trout, crab, and mussels. But oily fish are high in environmental pollutants, so limit your intake and favor smaller species (these toxins accumulate up the food chain).

192
Cut back on sugar

It's easy to remove bags of sugar from your cupboards, but hidden sugar lurks in a surprising number of savory and sweet foods. Check the labels of processed pies, savory snacks, conserves, condiments, and soft drinks.

193
Brown sugar

Although the nutritional value is the same, the browner the sugar the more flavor it has and so the less you need. You may find you prefer "raw" sugars such as muscovado or demerara to white refined sugar.

194
Try honey

Honey is sweeter than sugar, has fewer calories, and contains vitamins and minerals and plant nutrients that keep your cells healthy (darker honey, such as buckwheat, has a higher antioxidant content). Honey also enhances the growth of "good" bacteria in the gut. Many hay fever sufferers report that local honey helps them stay fit in the pollen season.

195
Portion distortion

A 2006 study monitoring young adults at a breakfast buffet found that they served themselves portions of cereal 25 percent greater than recommended. Download a portion-size card to remind everyone in your family what a portion looks like.

196
Top tips
A good store cupboard never runs out of healthy meals if it contains the following cans:
- Plum tomatoes
- Chick peas
- Kidney beans
- Mackerel
- Sardines
- Sweetcorn

197
Salty culprits
Processed foods tend to be higher in salt than homemade, accounting for 77 percent of the salt found in food. Opt for homemade when you can.

198
Alternatives to salt
High salt intake raises blood pressure, which increases risk of stroke and heart and kidney disease. Keep your spice and herb rack well stocked to cut the need for salt when cooking.

199
Buy a bread machine
To avoid huge amounts of salt and worrying additives in processed bread, bake your own the foolproof way with a bread machine. It takes the effort out of pizza dough, too.

200
Salt-free pizza topping
The only salt in this delicious pizza topping comes from the anchovies and black olives, which you can omit if you prefer.

201
Breton pancakes
These are great for incorporating milk and eggs into breakfast or dessert. The recipe uses buckwheat, which is an ancient grain traditional in Brittany, the home of crêpes.

- 2 cups plain flour
- ¾ buckwheat flour (*blé noir*)
- 1 tbsp demerara sugar
- 4 eggs, whisked
- 2 cups low-fat milk
- ¼ cup organic butter
- lemon and runny honey, to serve

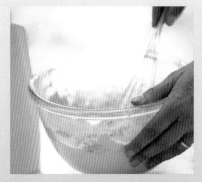
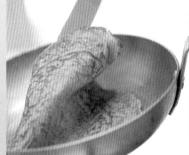
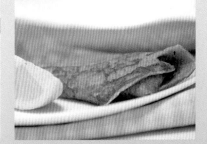

1 Combine the flours and sugar in a large bowl. Pour in the eggs. Stir to a stiff paste. Pour in the milk little by little, stirring constantly. Melt the butter and whisk in. Leave, covered, for two hours at room temperature.

2 Place a frying pan over high heat. Add a tiny pat of butter. Once melted, add a ladleful of mixture, tipping to distribute well. When the underside is light brown, toss to turn and cook the other side.

3 Squeeze over a good amount of lemon juice and a drizzle of honey. Roll up the pancake and serve while piping hot. Store any unused mixture in the fridge for use the following day.

4–6 onions, finely chopped
1–2 tbsp olive oil
1 x 15oz (425g) plum tomatoes, chopped
1 tsp freshly ground black pepper
good pinch of herbes de Provence
1oz (30g) anchovies in olive oil
1 tbsp capers, soaked
handful of black olives

Fry the onions in the olive oil over low heat until soft. Add the tomatoes and increase the heat, stirring until the juice has reduced. Spread the mixture over pizza bases (see No. 283), then scatter over the black pepper, herbs, anchovies, capers, and olives. Cook in a 400°F (200°C) oven until crispy, 12–15 minutes. Serves 4.

202
Fruit and veg in all forms
To ensure you always have some fruit and vegetables in, buy them canned, bottled, dried, and frozen.

203
Frozen nutrition
Invest in a chest freezer. Research from the Austrian Consumers Association found that vegetables picked in season and frozen retain more nutrients than produce flown in out of season.

204
Roast chickens
While it may sound surprising, many people don't know how to roast a chicken. Yet chicken is low in fat and calories and makes a hassle-free meal if you keep a free-range bird in the freezer and practice a roasting recipe. Serve with a salad, vegetables, rice, or couscous. The leftovers make a great low-fat sandwich filling. Make stock from the carcass for a nutritious soup.

205
Top bottled produce
Keep these in a cupboard to stir into pasta or make pizza toppings and increase your vegetable load after the grocery store is closed:

- Olives
- Sun-dried tomatoes
- Capers
- Anchovies
- Olive oil

206
Think grains
US nutritionists urge us to make grains 45-65 percent of our diet—that's wheat, rice, oats, corn, rye and barley (potatoes sit in this food group, too). UK recommendations make it about 50 percent. Can you fill at least half your pantry with these items?

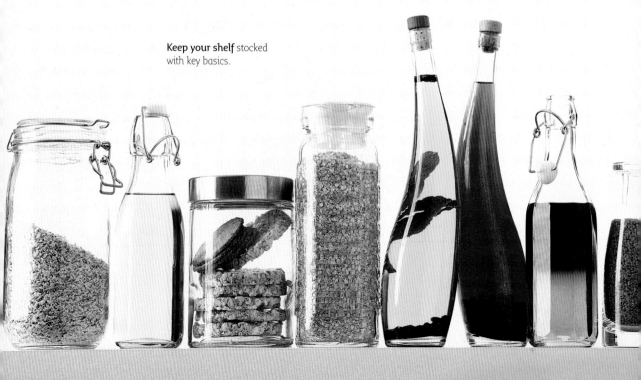

Keep your shelf stocked with key basics.

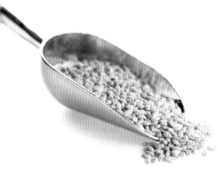

Can you fill at least half your food cupboards with different grains?

207
Whole is best

When stocking up on grains, look for "whole" or "unrefined" versions: they contain every part of a grain seed, including all its vitamins, minerals, and plant nutrients, plus the fiber that keeps you feeling full for longer. They keep your heart healthy and your weight in check.

208
Go organic

Favor organic whole grain products. When every part of the grain is used, it tends to carry pesticide residue. In a UK study, wholemeal bread was found to contain more residues than any other food.'

209
Fiber full

If you're over 65, you may need more fiber than when you were younger—from fruit, vegetables, and whole grains—and more water with it. Both ease constipation, which is thought to affect 20 percent of older people.

210
Try ancient grains

The grains humans ate before wheat came along are generally unrefined, higher in minerals than wheat, and very tasty. Look for spelt, kamut, amaranth, teff, quinoa, and millet. People who are wheat-sensitive may find them easier to digest.

211
Red fruit antioxidants

Don't store red-colored fruit—including tomatoes—in the fridge, because more cancer-defying antioxidants seem to develop in the flesh at room temperature.

To boost antioxidant levels, keep red fruits, including tomatoes, at room temperature.

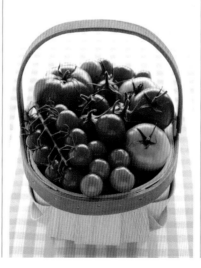

212
Add in pulses

Legumes, or pulses, count as one portion of fruit or vegetables, and are as good a source of fiber as bran (and a vital source of protein and iron for non-meat-eaters). Stock your pantry with dried and canned beans, lentils, and peas in their many varieties.

213
Chile heat

Capsaicin, the heating constituent of chiles, has been shown in several studies to boost heat generation, which causes us to burn more calories. It also reduces blood cholesterol. The hotter the chile, the more capsaicin.

214
Spices for metabolism

Spices stimulate digestion by stimulating enzymes in the pancreas and small intestine, and by increasing bile secretion (vital to digest and absorb fat). Black pepper, cardamom, clove, bay leaf, nutmeg, mace, fenugreek and cumin seeds, and dry ginger were found in a Tamil Nadu study to improve glucose and fat metabolism, while in a US Agricultural Research Service study, cinnamon regulated glucose metabolism and reduced blood-sugar, cholesterol, and triglyceride levels.

Grow your own

Growing some of your own produce benefits your body long before you put it in your mouth. Light gardening burns as many calories per hour as dancing or golf, and studies suggest gardeners tend to have a sunny outlook on life (depression and obesity go hand in hand). They also eat a greater variety of vegetables more often than non-gardeners.

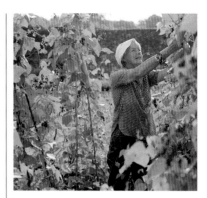

Be careful not to strain your neck when doing tasks that involve reaching up.

215
Get out early
If you can't fit in all the tasks you need to do on the weekend, get up half an hour early and tackle some jobs before work.

216
Nurture your mind
Researchers from Loughborough University in the UK found that horticulture offered a mental and emotional shape-up as well as physical toning. Being surrounded by trees and plants seems to reduce stress, muscle tension, and blood pressure, and offers an opportunity for relaxation and emotional release.

217
Warm-up
Avoid injury by easing yourself in with a warm-up before digging or bending over to weed: briskly walk around the garden, making a mental list of tasks that need to be done.

218
Garden circuit
Staying in one position for any length of time may lead to injury. Make yourself a mini circuit of tasks, and spend 10 minutes on each: weeding, pruning, digging, mowing, raking leaves, clipping. Briefly stretch between each one.

219
Alternate sides
To make gardening more of a workout, use your less favored hand and foot: put your left foot forward to rake, then your right, or place your least strong foot on the spade.

220
Make more trips
If you have heavy loads to carry, such as earthenware pots, make more trips with fewer objects. This saves your back and arms from injury and gives a longer cardio workout.

221
Reach out
Working with your arms above your head, such as pruning or clipping, works your heart strongly, but it can strain the neck, so take a rest and stretch after five minutes. You might like to divide a hedge into sections and clip one a day rather than trying to complete it all in one go.

222
Pull, don't carry
To save your back, roll heavy objects onto a tarp and drag them to their destination rather than carrying or lifting into a wheelbarrow.

223
Choosing a spade
Hard work such as turning compost or double-digging counts as a weights workout. You'll stay with the task longer if you have

good-quality tools. To preserve your posture, you may need a smaller-sized spade than you're used to, or one with a longer handle that allows you to stand upright rather than stooping. Try out a few at a garden center, choosing the lightest good-quality tool, and keep the blade sharp to minimize wasted effort.

224
Clever digging

Digging can stress the body. However, digging safely forces you to exercise the muscles in your arms and legs while protecting your back. **Stand directly** in front of the bed. Put in the blade close to your body. Step onto the top of the spade, bending at your knees and hips rather than rounding your back. **Keeping your back** neutral and chest wide, use your arms and shoulders to position the soil on the spade. **Keeping the load** as close to your body as possible (and to your center of gravity, your hips), pivot on one foot to cast the load to one side, always keeping it in front of you. Try not to twist your spine.

225
Make a raised bed

Essentially large planting boxes, raised beds are safer for gardeners who are prone to a bad back. If you use four pressure-treated railway sleepers (avoid those treated with creosote or chemical preservatives) to mark out the edges, you need no nails. This is a good winter job. **Mark out the area** you wish to cover using string attached to stakes; don't make it wider than you can comfortably reach. Dig over, removing turf, weeds, or plants. **Have the delivery man** position the sleepers on all four sides. **Fill with topsoil** and compost or other soil conditioner, such as well-rotted manure, seaweed, or leaf mold. On clay soil you may like to start with a 2in (5cm) gravel layer covered in sand. You're now ready to plant.

226
Garden together

In many countries, sales of vegetable seeds are now surpassing those of flowers. Can you plant produce in a community garden with a group of liked-minded people? This can make the work manageable for people with busy lives.

227
Online know-how

Need advice when frost gets your early potatoes or bugs reduce your cabbages to skeletons? Use an online support forum: www.growveg.com helps you design a vegetable patch, while www.gardenaction.co.uk offers a one-stop service on monthly tasks and pest-beating.

Develop a mini circuit as you work in the garden and spend 10 minutes on each task.

Easy to grow and a reliable fruiter, the blueberry can help lower levels of bad cholesterol.

228
What to grow

In a small plot, why not concentrate on fruit and vegetables you can't find in supermarkets—or can't afford? Perhaps unusual salad leaves, ruby chard, heirloom tomatoes, foods with an exceptional taste such as a fingerling potato variety or fiery chiles, or soft fruit that doesn't travel well, such as raspberries.

229
Raise blueberries

One of the easiest fruits to grow in a pot and a reliable fruiter even in cooler climates, blueberries contain compounds that are effective for lowering "bad" (LDL) cholesterol and other blood fats. Plant during the winter in a large pot filled with ericaceous soil; place in a sunny, sheltered spot and water well.

230
Planter potatoes

Buy seed potatoes in early spring and place in a dark, cool place for a few weeks until chitted (sprouted), then bury in a large planter with plenty of compost and well-rotted manure. As the leaves grow, rake the soil around them into a mound. They're ready when the white flowers appear.

231
Instant gardening

If you failed to grow your own vegetable plants from seed, don't give up on gardening and wallow in guilt and inactivity; order seedlings from an instant garden company that delivers ready-grown plants to your door, and try again.

232
Keep livestock

Once you feel competent growing a few vegetables, you might like to explore raising livestock. The easiest option is a few chickens—possible even in a small town garden—but some households opt to share the cost of raising a pig and the effort of caring for it. Mucking out, feeding, and watering will keep your figure trim as well as encourage your family to tune into where food comes from, and how, given the precious lives of animals, we should support good-quality meat over cheap, processed meals.

233
Post-gardening stretch

Stand in front of a (cleared) kitchen table so the tops of your thighs rest against the table edge and tiptoe your feet backward. Lie your whole upper body on the table, resting your head on your hands. Now gently relax your knees and legs, giving your lower back a soothing stretch. Rest here for 5 minutes.

Rearing chickens provides a home-grown food source of the most natural variety.

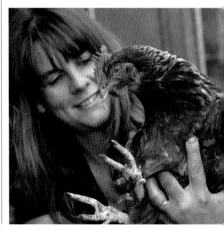

Shopping circuit

Venturing away from the supermarket can turn your shopping trip into a circuit-training session, with lots of walking, lifting, and carrying. But this type of shopping can be pleasurable too: the farmers' market, pick-your-own farms, and specialty delis are filled with healthy unprocessed items that make you fall in love with food, from artisan bread and cheese and local fruit and vegetables to home-cured meat and fish.

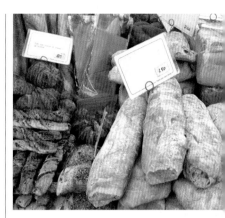

Traditional bread not only tastes better but is easier to digest than a supermarket loaf.

234
Know the truth

Why are healthy, unprocessed foods invisible in supermarkets? The answer is because they don't profit food manufacturers. The number of packaged foods available in the US is up to more than a quarter of a million compared with an unchanged number of "traditional foods." Choose where your money goes and buy healthy foods.

235
Shop locally

What foods are available within walking distance of your home or work? Is there a farm shop, a weekly market, a seafood van, or local bakery? Walk there when you can.

236
Try the farmers' market

A farmers' market is less of a chore than a fun morning out: you can ask the producers for cooking tips, sample delicacies, and above all buy delicious raw ingredients. The people who produce this food also keep the fields, hedgerows, and marine environment looking good enough to tempt you out for country walks—another reason to keep them in business.

237
Use a backpack

Take a lightweight backpack on shopping trips: evenly distributing the weight you carry protects your back, and is a weight-training method used by athletes.

238
Order organic

Eating a wide variety of foods maximizes nutrition and minimizes intolerances. Have an organic produce box delivered weekly for a constantly changing roster of ingredients, from asparagus and purple sprouting broccoli to soft fruit and fresh peas. Many are available locally for only a few weeks of the year and some are heritage varieties not available in supermarkets.

239
Artisan baking

Do you have a local "craft" baker who uses time-honored baking ingredients and methods? Their loaves not only taste better, but long fermentation seems to make them easier to digest, especially for those with wheat sensitivities. These loaves also tend to have a chewy crust, which exercises the jaw.

240
Eat fair

Staying in shape mentally means feeling good about the way you live. An easy way to do this is to buy

Fruit picked locally retains a high proportion of minerals and vitamins.

fairly traded foods, which give producers a fair wage and support educational and healthcare projects that improve the lives of others in the community.

241
Pick-your-own

In summer, enjoy an afternoon out at a pick-your-own farm, harvesting ripe fruit that doesn't travel well, such as berries, apples, and plums.

242
Hedgerow harvesting

In the past, blackberries, hazelnuts, and mushrooms came from the hedgerow and forest floor, not the supermarket. They're still there if you look for them. Enjoy the walking, climbing, and stretching—and the calming influence of roaming outdoors in fresh air.

243
Hedgerow crumble

You can substitute seasonal fruit for the apples and blackberries in this recipe—tart rhubarb and gooseberries taste delicious.

3½ cups blackberries
2 cups cored and sliced apples
1½ tbsp muscovado (brown) sugar
½ cup butter, straight from the fridge
½ cup wholemeal flour
5 tbsp jumbo oats
2 tbsp hazelnuts, crushed
1½ tbsp pumpkin seeds

Heat the oven to 350°F (180°C). Place the fruit at the bottom of a pie dish with 1 tbsp of the sugar. In a bowl, cut the butter into pieces and rub into the flour until the mixture resembles coarse breadcrumbs, then stir in the oats, hazelnuts, seeds, and remaining sugar. Moisten with 2 tsp water. Pile the crumble topping over the fruit and bake for 30 minutes, or until lightly browned on top.

Reshape your shop

When you have to hit the supermarket, try to avoid the highly processed foods that often include ingredients linked with obesity and heart disease, such as high-fructose corn syrup (HFCS), trans-fats, and added salt and sugar. People who consume food and drinks high in added sugar tend to consume more calories than those who eat home-cooked meals.

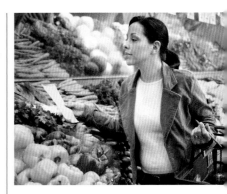

Challenge yourself to take a list shopping and come home with nothing extra!

244
Take a list
Before the weekly grocery shop, plan at least five healthy meals and list the ingredients. Can you come home with nothing extra?

245
Cruise the margins
In supermarkets, stick to the perimeters, where the least packaged food is stacked: milk and eggs, fresh fruit and vegetables, unprepared fish and meat, and bread. Make strategic dashes into the brightly lit central aisles for red wine, olive oil, rice, and toiletries.

246
Limit shopping time
Limit the amount of time you spend in the supermarket to avoid temptation. Try shopping 30 minutes before the store closes or during your lunch hour. Bulk-buy staples monthly (toilet paper, toothpaste, low-fat milk, and whole grain loaves to freeze), visiting greengrocers and butchers' shops between trips.

247
Try something new
On each shopping trip, buy one fruit you've never tried and one new vegetable. At market stalls or delis, ask how you might cook it. Challenge your kids to Google a recipe for it.

248
Cut out trans-fats
Trans-fats are a product of food processing (hydrogenation). They have no nutritional value and damage the heart. Keep your consumption low by avoiding ready-made cakes, cookies, pies, and margarine.

249
Read the list
It's easy to cut back on processed food: just don't buy anything with more than five ingredients or a list that reads like a science equation. The least processed foods—fresh fruit and vegetables, meat and fish, milk, olive oil—have no ingredients lists.

250
Spotlight data
To simplify the nutritional labels on packages, ignore everything except the saturated fat and sugar content. If either have more than 4g per serving, put it back.

251
Is low-fat healthier?
More and more food manufacturers claim product ranges to be "low-fat" or "sugar-free." But some of the ingredients used to replace the fat and sugar might be less healthy than the butter and sugar we are trying to avoid. There may even be more sugar, salt, or fat than in the regular equivalent. To stay in shape, it's best to avoid these foods.

252
Variety, variety

Different types of vegetables are rich in different nutrients, so include some from all these groups in your cart: dark green (broccoli, spinach), orange and red (carrots, sweet potatoes, tomatoes, peppers), pulses (chick peas, lentils), starchy vegetables (potatoes, peas)—then look for others that don't fit the categories, including salad ingredients and mushrooms.

253
Increase-decrease

When you increase the number of nutrient-dense products in your basket (milk, yogurt, whole grains, vegetables) try to decrease the amount of nutrient-free products you buy (soft drinks, processed pies, sweets) rather than picking up another basket or a bigger cart.

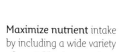

Maximize nutrient intake by including a wide variety of vegetables in your shop.

254
Spotting sugar

The following are all forms of sugar in disguise: sucrose, glucose, dextrose, fructose, maltose, corn sweetener, (high-fructose) corn syrup, malt syrup, molasses, syrup, invert syrup, honey, fruit juice concentrates. Avoid these sugars when you can.

255
Avoid corn syrup

High-fructose corn syrup (HFCS) is a new sweetener used to stick other ingredients together, and our bodies haven't evolved a mechanism to handle it, argues food polemicist Michael Pollan. It has been linked to obesity and high triglyceride levels, a risk factor for heart disease. Look for it in ingredients lists and avoid.

256
Artificial sweeteners

Numerous studies report side effects with sweeteners, from headaches to digestive problems. More research is needed, but some people prefer to avoid them.

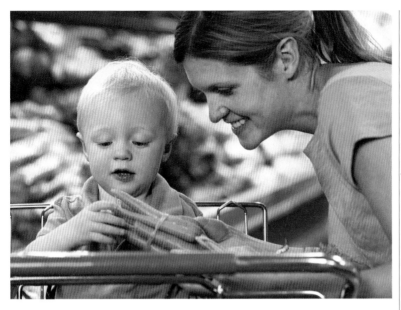

Buy different types of vegetables at the store to ensure a wide range of nutrients.

257
Don't be fooled

One US study found that of 37 foods featuring fruit prominently on the package, 51 percent contained no actual fruit! Check the ingredients list before you buy.

258
Spotting salt

To spot hidden salt, look for the words "sodium chloride" on labels. Choose products containing no more than 0.6g salt per 100g.

259
Compare products

Salt levels in the same type of foods, such as store-bought soups, vary enormously. In particular, carefully compare labels of economy brands, and also organic soups.

260
Think about soy

Soy is added to many processed foods, but it mimics estrogen, and excessive intake has been linked with hormone disruption and immunity, thyroid, fertility, and developmental issues. Limit your consumption.

261
Makes uS Greedy?

The flavor enhancer monosodium glutamate MSG (E621) found in many snack foods, such as flavored crisps, may interfere with appetite regulation (making us want to eat more). It has also been linked with headaches, heart palpitations, asthma, and nausea. If you eat chips, stick to salted, which contain nothing but oil, potatoes, and salt.

262
Colorings

The following artificial food colorings in combination with the preservative sodium benzoate (E211) have been linked with hyperactivity and behavioral problems in children: sunset yellow (E110), quinoline yellow (E104), carmoisine (E122), allura red (E129), tartrazine (E102), and ponceau 4R (E124). Check sweets, soft drinks, colored icing, and ice cream before buying.

263
Look organic

Organic processed foods, from cookies to chips, contain fewer additives, which makes them a better choice than regular processed foods.

264
Go green

To increase your motivation to reduce your reliance on processed food, think green. Processed food increases your carbon footprint because it tends to be highly packaged: 60 percent of household waste is packaging.

Cooking from scratch

The US, Scandinavia, UK, and Japan are kings of the packaged food market—and the trend is set to grow in Western Europe as well as emerging Eastern European markets. The rise in popularity of packaged food is echoed by a decline in cooking skills and food traditions such as the family meal—all blamed for the obesity crisis. Teach yourself to cook one dish this week and join a cooking renaissance that will make you thinner and happier.

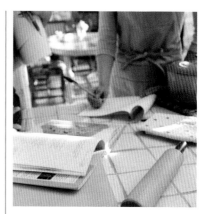

Plan what you eat on a regular basis to help you keep your healthy diet on track.

265

Eat the seasons

If you cook using fresh produce, you can make the most of seasonal ingredients. Many natural therapists believe that eating with the seasons makes it more likely that you will take in the nutrients your body needs: comforting carbohydrate-rich root vegetables in winter may help to lift seasonal depression, and many summer fruits rehydrate the body. Locally picked foods, which have traveled less distance, may be higher in vitamin C, which degrades in storage.

266

Make a meal planner

This helps you keep track of what you're eating—how many fruits and vegetables, how much oily fish—and streamlines your shopping and helps you think ahead, so you can prepare meals when you have more time. Spend a night in with some cookbooks or the Internet and mark recipes you enjoy. Repeat four times a year at the start of each season.

267

The art of list making

Once you've compiled a meal planner, list the ingredients you need for each dish on a master shopping list; key them into an online grocery order so you never lack healthy essentials.

268

Gourmet weekend

If you don't have time in the week, be a weekend cook and supersize dishes to freeze in portions for busy days.

269

Slow cooking

Join a local Slow Cooking *convivium*, a group who meets to celebrate simple ingredients, local producers, and the joy of socializing with food. The movement started in Italy in 1986 as an antidote to the fast-food joints and processed food the founders believed were eating up their ancient culinary culture.

270

Quick fish

Fresh fish is the ultimate quick meal. Buy from a fish market, (have them fillet it), then grill for a few minutes

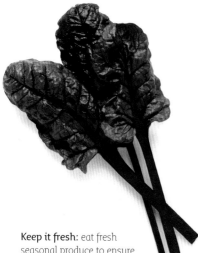

Keep it fresh: eat fresh seasonal produce to ensure maximum nutrient intake.

on each side, or wrap in tin foil with herbs and a squeeze of lemon and bake for 20 minutes in a hot oven.

271
One-pot cooking

It can be hard to find huge stockpots (5 quarts or larger) in the stores, so shop online for one perfect for slow cooking. Cast iron casseroles hold heat and so need little energy. Throw in some root vegetables and stock with some browned stewing meat at lunchtime on a slow simmer and by evening you will have a delicious stew. It will taste even better the next day, once the flavors have melded.

272
Steam it

To preserve the greatest amount of nutrients in cooked vegetables, steam them. Look for a steamer with a lid that fits snugly inside a pan.

273
Meat treat

Meat consumption has increased five-fold in the last 50 years, yet meat and dairy foods contribute the greatest amount of saturated fat to our diet, increasing the risk of obesity, type 2 diabetes, heart disease, and some cancers. By cutting down on meat, you eat more fruits and vegetables. Reducing the amount of meat in your diet may also protect against osteoporosis, to keep you exercising safely into older age, found researchers from Cornell University.

274
Flavor enhancer

In many traditional food cultures, red meat is a treat enjoyed on feast days or used in small amounts to flavor dishes based on nutrition-packed vegetables and fruit, and filling whole grains and pulses. Experts believe this may be the healthiest way to eat meat.

Meat, veggies, and stock all in one pot make an easy, nutritious, and delicious meal.

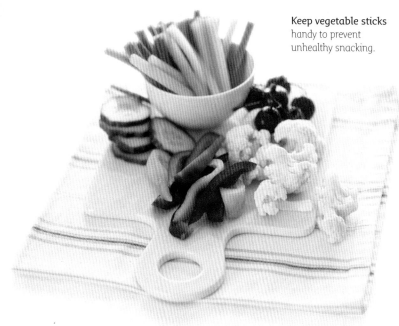

Keep vegetable sticks handy to prevent unhealthy snacking.

275
Rest your body

Enjoy the benefits of a vegetarian diet—lower average body weight and reduced rates of heart disease, stroke, and type 2 diabetes—by building meatless days into your week.

276
Don't snack and cook

If you're tempted to eat the ingredients as you cook, keep some vegetable sticks in the fridge and snack on these to keep you going.

277
The lean bin

A study from the University of Arizona in Tucson found that 40–50 percent of food is discarded. In the UK, it's every third bag of shopping carried home. Don't let your resolution to eat more fruit and vegetables go with them: juice over-ripe fruit or blend into milkshakes, make sauces with produce about to blow, such as tomatoes or apples and pears, and refrigerate or freeze.

278
Bean and sausage casserole

This spicy casserole is light on meat but heavy on flavor.

18oz (500g) bag assorted pulses (e.g., cannellini, kidney, garbanzo beans)
2 tbsp olive oil
4 onions, peeled and roughly chopped
2 red peppers, seeded and chopped
8 cloves garlic, thinly sliced
2 tsp herbes de Provence
1 tbsp ground cumin
1 x 15oz (425g) plum tomatoes, chopped
1 tbsp Worcestershire sauce
1 tbsp sweet (dulce) Spanish paprika
black pepper and sea salt, to taste
4 spicy sausages

Soak the pulses overnight. Drain and rinse well. Place in a large pan and cover with water (do not salt). Bring to a boil and allow to boil for 10 minutes, then simmer (covered) for 75 minutes, until just soft.
Heat the oil in a large saucepan and fry the onions and peppers on low heat until soft, about 20 minutes. Add the garlic, herbs, and cumin and heat through for 5 minutes. Add the tomatoes, Worcestershire sauce, paprika, and seasoning, and cook until reduced slightly, about 10 minutes.
Add the beans and cooking liquid to cover. Bring to a simmer, then turn the heat to low, cover, and let it bubble for 2 hours. Add more Worcestershire sauce, paprika, or herbs, to taste. Fry the sausages until browned on all sides, cut into slices, and stir into the pan just before serving. Serves 4–6.

279
Fruit for dessert

In the Mediterranean region, everyday dessert is fruit rather than a cooked, calorie-laden dish. Think likewise. The traditional Mediterranean way of eating, rich in fresh and dried fruit and vegetables, seems to protect against excessive weight gain and promote longevity.

Kitchen workout

If it weren't for processed food, we'd spend more time (and calories) beating, stirring, and whisking. The more active you are in the kitchen, the more you can eat without putting on weight, and so the more nutrients you're likely to encounter in a day.

280
Unplug the microwave

The growth in ready-made meals is underpinned by a love of microwave ovens in the US, UK, Japan, and Canada. Check how much more active you are in the kitchen if you turn off your microwave for a week.

281
Use a pestle and mortar

One of most effective pieces of kitchen gym equipment, a pestle and mortar, releases more flavorful compounds in food than a metal-bladed blender, which can leave watery ingredients, such as herbs, rather mushy. Buy the largest bowl and widest-headed pestle you can afford. When grinding, keep your wrist still, keeping the circular rotation in the arm and shoulder, and allow the circling action to do the work rather than sheer pressure. Give hard spices, such as black pepper, a stiff thump to break them before beginning to grind.

282
Kneading masterclass

Making bread by hand is a therapeutic way to keep active in the evening: even gentle continuous activity prompts the release of endorphins in the brain, bringing on a natural high, and touch of many kinds reduces levels of stress hormones. Knead the bread with your whole body: stand tall as you work, taking long, deep breaths that expand your abdomen, and move your body from your shoulders. As the dough becomes springier after about 10 minutes' kneading, notice whether knots in your shoulders and neck feel less tight.

Kneading therapy: keep active in the evening by making bread.

283

Pizza dough

This pizza base is light, crispy, and quite delicious!

1½oz (15g) dried yeast
¾ cup white bread flour
1¼ cups whole grain bread flour
½ tsp sea salt, finely ground
¼ cup olive oil
1 large egg, beaten
cornmeal, for sprinkling
olive oil for oiling

Put the yeast in a bowl and cover with 4 tbsp tepid water. Mix the flours and salt in a large bowl, then pour in the oil and egg and the frothy yeast mixture. Stir until well combined and the dough forms a pliable mass.

Knead for 10 minutes on a surface sprinkled with the cornmeal. Place in an oiled bowl and cover with a clean dish towel. Leave somewhere warm to rise until doubled in size (about 1½–2 hours).

Punch the dough to knock out the air, let it rest for 10 minutes, knead lightly, then roll out to the size of your baking pans. Add topping (see No. 200) and bake in a preheated 400°F (200°C) oven until crispy (about 20–25 minutes). Serves 4.

284

Ditch the food processor

It's more meditative to cream together butter and sugar by hand. Use this as an exercise in mindfulness when cooking a birthday cake: as you use elbow grease, think about what you love about the person you're baking for, and stir love into the mix!

285

How to cream

Make sure the ingredients are at room temperature. Put the butter in a mixing bowl and beat with the

286

Pesto by hand

The Italian fresh basil sauce pesto Genovese is traditionally made by hand using a pestle and mortar. This is a job older children love to take charge of.

- 2 bunches fresh basil
- 2 cloves garlic
- good pinch of coarse sea salt
- 2 tbsp pine nuts
- freshly ground black pepper, to taste
- 2 tbsp pecorino or Parmesan cheese, or half and half, coarsely grated
- 1–2 tbsp extra-virgin olive oil

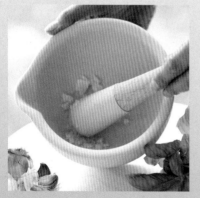

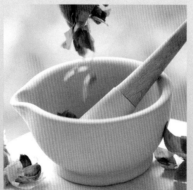

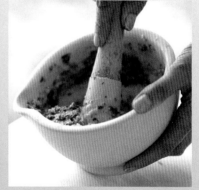

1 Remove the basil leaves from the stalks. If large, tear them (don't cut with a knife). Place the garlic and salt in the mortar and pound to a paste.

2 Slowly add the leaves, crushing to a thick-textured paste. Add the pine nuts, black pepper, and cheese, and grind until well amalgamated.

3 Finally, mix in the oil until you have a consistency you like. Stir into cooked pasta or use as a topping for baked potatoes or grilled fish.

wooden spoon to soften. Pour in the sugar and beat for 8–10 minutes—the aim is to add tiny air bubbles that cause the mixture to rise when heated—think of each one as a bubble of love! Swap hands, but keep beating in the same direction. The mix is ready for the eggs and flour when light, fluffy, and pale.

287
Move around
Standing in one position for too long causes blood to pool in the lower body and can fatigue the muscles. Try to move around as you cook and wash dishes to encourage blood flow to the feet, or do calf raises as you stand: rise onto the balls of your feet, feeling a contraction in your calves, then gradually lower your heels.

288
Wear soft shoes
Standing on hard kitchen floors in heels or barefoot can cause foot pain; when cooking or cleaning, wear soft cushioned shoes such as sneakers or Birkenstocks.

289
Stretch out
If you have a strong bar in your kitchen, grab it with your hands shoulder-width apart and walk your feet back until your legs and back make a right angle. Bend your knees a little, taking your weight in your arms; this is a wonderful stretch for your shoulders and back.

290
Wash dishes by hand
Washing dishes is one of the most time-consuming of household chores, and consequently burns a gratifying number of calories if you do it by hand—a 2006 survey suggested it burns more calories than floor-scrubbing or changing bed linen. If you're not convinced, wear a heart-rate monitor while you wash, stack, dry, and put away, and then compare to a session at the gym.

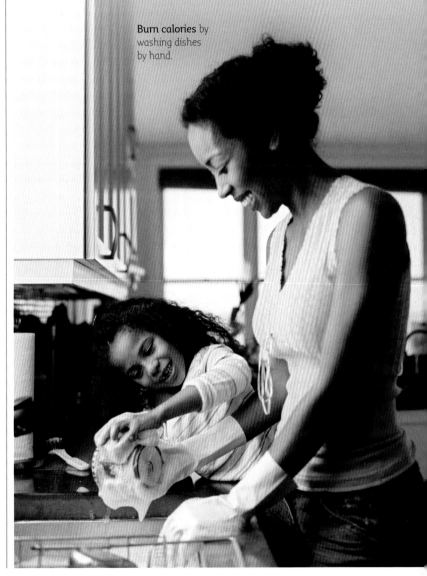

Burn calories by washing dishes by hand.

Around the table

Where and how we eat has surprisingly far-reaching consequences for our health and body shape. Studies suggest that people who prepare and eat food with family or friends eat better-balanced meals and a greater variety of healthy foods. American studies have found that children who eat meals regularly with their families have a better diet than those who don't—and they take it with them into adulthood.

291
Make time to share

In our increasingly busy lives, getting an entire household together for a meal takes determination. Try to schedule in a family meal two or three times a week, even if it means leaving work a little earlier or recording favorite TV programs. If evening meals are difficult, share a Saturday brunch or Sunday lunch.

292
Reduce the stress

Stress at mealtimes may contribute to obesity in children, state some pediatricians, so try to keep things calm: mealtimes aren't the place to tackle "issues." If you struggle, ask each family member to write down words they associate with meals, listing negatives (boring, arguments, smoky) in one column and positives (jokes, yummy, dessert) in another. Brainstorm ways you can get from one to the other.

293
Light some candles

Candlelight makes any meal an occasion and creates an inviting atmosphere of calmness, especially if you can't eat until late because of work or a long commute.

294
Turn that thing off

Families who turn off the TV while dining eat more nutritious foods than those who eat together with the TV on, found University of Minnesota researchers.

295
Saying grace

Giving thanks for food before eating is common to every religious tradition: in Jewish belief, this *berachah* also shows how we differ from the animals, who greedily start to gobble the moment food is put in front of them.

296
Non-denominational grace

"May the love around this table nourish our spirits, and inspire us to live in peace, hope, and joy, today and forever. Amen."

Light candles at the dinner table to create a calm and relaxing atmosphere.

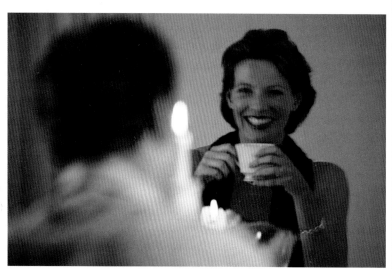

297
Yogic grace

Before eating, sit quietly, close your eyes, and tune in with yourself, watching your breathing become slower and deeper and relaxing areas of tension for two minutes. If it feels right, hold hands with others around the dinner table as you do so.

298
No seconds

Helping yourself to seconds can double the portion—and calories—you eat at dinner. Rather than dishing out food at the table, plate meals up elsewhere, and put leftovers into a freezer dish for days when you have less time to cook.

299
Savor the scents

The digestive process begins as soon as we smell a dish, so don't rush to start eating. Spending a few moments enjoying the scent prompts the mouth to produce saliva to lubricate food and ease swallowing.

300
How to chew

Many of us don't chew our food well enough to stimulate full digestion. Try to chew each mouthful 15–20 times before swallowing; this allows enzymes in

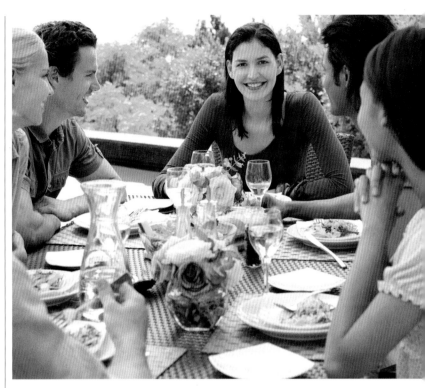

Sharing meals with family or friends is associated with eating a better-balanced diet.

the saliva to begin breaking down the food and causes the release of chemical signals to prepare the stomach lining, pancreas, and small intestines to kick into action.

301
20-minute dining

Signals of being full take about 20 minutes to pass from stomach to brain, so try to make a meal last 20 minutes. The monks of Mount Athos, Greece, are believed to have the world's healthiest diet—they have a bell that rings 20 minutes after the start of a meal, and whether finished or not, they leave the table.

302
Take a breather

After taking a mouthful, put down cutlery and focus on the food. Try to find words to describe the taste and textures; think about where the food came from and how it arrived at your plate. Pick up your fork only after the food has changed in texture and is small enough to swallow.

303
Leave the leftovers

If you're tempted to pick at leftovers when cleaning up, have someone else clear plates straight into the garbage.

Reshape your wardrobe

What you wear flags your body shape and state of mind to the world, so it really matters that your clothes fit and flatter. But American research shows that many of us keep two or more sets of clothing to cover our fluctuating size. To help keep weight loss permanent, clear out the supersized skeletons in your wardrobe—this could be the first step toward finding a new you.

304
Assess your wardrobe
Do you grade your wardrobe by size—size 14s to the left; 18-plus to the right? You're giving yourself an excuse not to keep eating healthily—it's like keeping a secret sugar stash in your kitchen. Make a date in your diary this week for a clear-out.

305
Buy a tape measure
Keep a tape measure in your closet. If your waist measures 32in for women and 37in for men (36in for smaller men), you have a raised risk of heart attack, stroke, and diabetes. The risk is greatest if it measures over 35in for women or

Have a tape measure handy to keep track of your waist measurements.

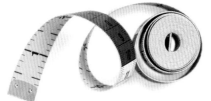

40in for men: go and see your doctor and adopt some of the strategies in this book.

306
What fits now?
Sort through your closet piece by piece. Make three piles: "fat" clothes, "skinny" clothes, and those that fit. Hang the last pile in your closet: look how much more room there is! Now ditch the first pile—with your new eating and exercise regime, you won't need them anytime soon. Don't put them into storage just in case. Can you take back those that still have their tags, eBay any, or take quality garments to a designer sale shop?

307
Skinny clothes
Look at the pile of clothes in your wardrobe that are reserved for skinny days. Realistically, how many will you wear again—how many of these are even in style or suit your

current lifestyle and age? Have a thorough clear-out, and hang only classic pieces that still flatter—and can fit—back in your wardrobe.

308
Don't go baggy
Wearing clothes that are too big for you doesn't hide excess pounds: it makes you look bigger than you are. Fitted clothes are much more flattering, slimming your silhouette, and emphasizing a womanly hour-glass figure.

309
Reading labels
In the last few years, high-end fashion sizing has gone haywire, with shops downgrading sizes to appeal to our size-0 aspirations. What was once size 12 may now be an 8; you may fit in a 10 in one store, but a 16 in another. Don't worry; just look for clothes made in France and Italy, where sizes (38 (small), 40, 42, 44 (extra large), relate to body measurements. German pattern cutting is similarly accurate, but sized slightly larger.

310
Wardrobe scenting
Essential oil of black pepper peps you up and is famed for its fat-busting properties; grapefruit lifts the spirits when you feel jaded, both

good qualities to cultivate when getting dressed. After clearing out your wardrobe, wet dust it, adding 4 drops of each oil to the final rinse water (wear rubber gloves).

311
Clothes-swap get together

Spend an evening swapping clothes with a girlfriend. Try on lots of different garments, then ask your friend to pick out an outfit she thinks suits the new you, then you do the same for her.

312
Emphasize your assets

Playing up your best parts is the key to distracting attention from parts of the body you're not so happy with. A great bust deserves plunging v-necks or a wrap dress; emphasize long legs by wearing skinny jeans with heels; and flatter a tiny waist with an attention-grabbing wide, cinched belt.

Swap clothes with friends and find new outfits to suit the new you.

313
Clothes for bloated days

If before your period you tend to bloat, keep a pair of high-waisted flared trousers or a skirt and a long-line jacket that covers your bottom and thighs in your wardrobe.

314
Value your underwear

Stand in front of the mirror in your underwear. Do your bra straps dig in? Do you bulge over your cups? Does your chest merge into your waist? When underwear fits well, your clothes look better.

315
Getting measured

If you haven't been measured for a bra in the last year, visit a lingerie boutique or department store. Specialists will conjure up a garment that changes the way you think about your shape forever. A good bra also encourages you to walk tall, with chest open and shoulders back and down, which can also reduce neck and shoulder pain.

316
Shapewear

Support underwear that flattens the tummy and lifts the buttocks can be a lifesaver beneath clinging dresses on special occasions.

317
Exercise wear

If you don't feel happy in exercise gear, you're unlikely to keep exercise up. Invest in clothes that flatter and make you feel confident, matching them to the activity and what others are wearing. For yoga and exercise classes, choose garments that stretch with you but allow the teacher to see your form to correct your posture. For outside activity, wear enough layers to counter changing weather conditions—rain, sun, wind—which might include gloves and a hat.

318
Flower essences for the mirror

If you hate looking in the mirror, these remedies may bring courage. Place 4 drops in water and sip until symptoms subside.
- Crab Apple (Bach): if you are unable to accept your physical imperfections, and assume others won't either.
- Chrysanthemum (Californian): remedy for those mourning lost youth and afraid of aging.
- Pretty Face (Californian): if you feel "ugly" or over-identify with your appearance.

Choose exercise clothes appropriate for the activity, but which also fit and flatter your shape.

A night in the bathroom

You can make an enormous difference to the way you feel about your shape by spending the occasional evening spoiling yourself in the bathroom, emerging with newly softened skin, a glowing complexion, and shiny, swinging locks. When you feel this good, you stand taller and smile more often: the instant way to transform your shape and sense of well-being.

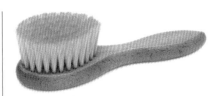

Stimulate circulation and exfoliation with a brisk dry-brushing session before a bath.

319
Salt and pepper scrub
The salt in this body scrub sloughs off dead skin cells to leave your skin feeling smooth while the oil imparts a sheen.

2 tbsp sea salt, finely ground
1 tsp freshly ground black pepper, finely milled
2 tbsp runny honey
1 tbsp olive oil

Mix together the salt and pepper in a bowl, then stir in the honey and olive oil. Massage handfuls over damp skin from heels to shoulders, always in the direction of the heart. Rinse off in a cool shower.

320
Cellulite scrub
To counter cellulite, add 2 drops each of fresh essential oils of rosemary and cypress to half the salt and pepper scrub above. After pummeling your buttocks and thighs with your fists (keep your wrists soft), massage with the scrub, making firm, circular strokes in the direction of your heart. Rinse off in the bath or shower. (Avoid if you are pregnant or have epilepsy or high blood pressure.)

321
Bottom-shaping bridge
While you wait for the bath to fill, sit on the floor with your hands behind you and feet hip-width apart. As you inhale, tighten your bottom and push your hips to the ceiling—take the pubic bone as high as you can. Lower your hips to the floor, keeping your bottom tight. Relax before repeating.

322
Cold-jet treatment
To target areas of cellulite, after a shower use the shower head to give the thighs, buttocks, and abdomen a bracing blast, moving the jet in small circles and taking the water as cool as you dare. Rub dry vigorously with a waffle towel.

323
Dry brushing
Use a body brush on dry skin before a bath to stimulate circulation and exfoliation. Use quick back-and-forth strokes up the body from the soles of the feet to the top of the shoulders and then up your arms, working toward your heart. Stroke gently over the underarm area to stimulate the lymphatic system. Avoid delicate areas such as the chest.

324
Oatmeal skin scrubber
Use as a stimulating alternative to soap if you have delicate skin.

6 tbsp fine oatmeal
6 tbsp dried rose petals, crushed

Pile the ingredients in the center of a piece of muslin and tie to secure. Float in the tub while the tap is running; use as a soap substitute.

325
Blue bath
Color therapists believe that bathing in colored water positively affects

body and mind. Research shows that being surrounded by blue can reduce the appetite and that exposure to blue light decreases blood pressure and heart rate. In the evening, tint your bath a restful shade of blue with blue bath salts. This is thought to ease insomnia, too.

326
Improving skin tone
The following tissue salts may be recommended by homeopaths. They are taken in the same way as other homeopathic remedies.
- Calc. Fluor: boosts elasticity

of the skin and blood vessels, helping to prevent stretch marks and varicose veins.
- Silica: for healing skin abrasions, dry patches, and eczema.
- Nat. Mur.: for rebalancing water in the tissues, preventing dehydration of the skin and high blood pressure, which can contribute to broken veins.

327
Garam masala bath bag
This fragrant blend of spices contains a number of antioxidant ingredients reputed to boost metabolism.

1 tsp black peppercorns, crushed
1 tbsp cardamoms, crushed
1 tsp cumin seeds
1 tbsp cloves
4 drops essential oil of coriander

Pile all the ingredients into a piece of muslin, drop over the essential oil, and tie to secure. Float beneath the hot tap while running a warm bath.

328
Arm shaping
Try this after a bath to work the triceps at the backs of the arms. Make sure your hands and the sides of the bath are completely dry.

329
Honey facial clay
This clay facial draws impurities from the skin while also replenishing it by imparting minerals and trace elements to leave the complexion feeling taut and fresh.

- 1 egg yolk
- 2 tsp runny honey
- 1 tsp grapeseed oil
- 1 vitamin E capsule
- 1 tbsp bentonite clay
- 3–5 tbsp rosewater

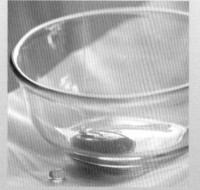

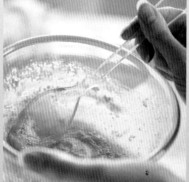

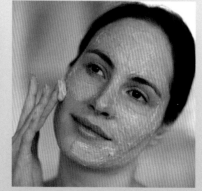

1 In a bowl, stir the egg yolk, honey, and oil together well. Prick the capsule and squeeze the contents into the mixture.

2 Mix in the clay little by little until you have a thick paste. Use enough of the rosewater to give a consistency you prefer.

3 Apply to cleansed skin, avoiding the eye area. Relax for 15 minutes. Wipe away with a warm, wet cloth, then splash with tepid water.

Place your palms on each side of the bath with your feet in front of you, hip-width apart, so your body drops in a straight line from ear to hips. Breathing out, bend your arms to lower your body. Don't take the weight on your feet; feel the backs of your arms supporting you. Go as low as you can. Inhaling, press on your palms and straighten your arms to raise your body. Don't cheat by using your legs. Repeat up to 15 times. Work up to 3 sets.

330

Rosemary rinse

After washing, give your hair extra shine with an herbal rinse: place a rosemary tea bag in a mug and pour over just-boiled water. Steep for 15-20 minutes, then use as a final rinse.

331

Scalp massage

Massage stimulates blood circulation to the scalp, leaving you feeling both more relaxed and energized and can add body to lacklustre locks. You will need a little grapeseed oil. Warm the oil by standing the bottle in a bowl of hot water. Pour a little into the palm of one hand, then rub your hands together to distribute it. Place your fingertips at your hairline, little fingers at the center,

thumbs by your temples. Keeping your fingers stiff, knuckles bent, make small circles that move the tissue beneath the surface of the skin. Move back an inch and repeat. Repeat up to your crown, then down to the nape of your neck. Work your thumbs into knotted muscles there. Finally, place your knuckles at the base of the skull and rotate.

332

Hair tugging

To increase circulation to hair follicles after washing your hair or before styling, grasp a handful of hair at the roots at the hairline above your eyes. Twist around your fingers, then tug. Move up to the crown then down to the nape of your neck. Shake out any tension in your hands.

333

Aloe hair mask

For hair that swings the next day, apply this nourishing hair mask half an hour before going to bed.

1 aloe vera leaf or 1 tbsp aloe gel
1 tbsp conditioner to suit your hair type
4 drops essential oil of ylang ylang
1 very ripe peeled and mashed banana
1 tbsp coconut milk

Score the aloe leaf and force out the gel with the back of a spoon, or squirt the gel from the tube. Stir into the conditioner, then add the essential oil. Mix in the banana and coconut milk. Massage into dry hair, from the roots down. Pile your hair up, cover with a shower cap, then wrap in a warmed towel for 20 minutes. Shower off, then wash and condition your hair as usual.

Put the swing back into your hair by applying an aloe vera hair mask before bed.

Detox your body

Every day our lungs, skin, liver, gut, and colon work hard to clear out the toxins that make us feel out of shape. However, detox diets, supplements, and remedies don't speed up this process—what keeps the detox organs functioning well is a good diet, plenty of exercise, and good hydration, as well as a few early nights and days off from alcohol. This is also the best way to detox after a period of indulgence.

334

Water flush

One of the best ways to help your kidneys process toxins is to drink enough water—around 6 to 8 glasses daily, and more in hotter climates. This is especially important when exercising—keep well hydrated by drinking water before and after a training session.

Drink plenty of water to keep your body well hydrated.

335

Cut back on alcohol

It takes 36 hours for your liver to rid your body of alcohol. Help it along by keeping well hydrated and by having a few alcohol-free days each week to give your detox organs a rest.

336

How much do you drink?

Most people underestimate the amount of alcohol they drink. Medical experts consider moderate use to be up to one drink a day for women and two for men—a drink is defined as 12fl oz beer, 5fl oz wine, or 1.5oz of spirits, which all contain around .54oz of alcohol. Drinking more than this may risk harming your health and adds unnecessary calories to your daily intake.

337

How large is your glass?

Just as food plate and portions have increased in the last 20 years, so have wine glasses and levels of alcohol in drinks. To stay in shape, use smaller glasses at home and check the alcohol content on the bottle. Regular beer has an alcohol content of 4-5%, table wine 9–12% and spirits 72%, but many popular drinks contain higher levels of alcohol—and more calories.

338
Watch out women

Alcohol harms women's bodies more than men's: women are lighter, smaller, and carry less water; they also have fewer enzymes that break down alcohol, resulting in greater organ damage.

339
Fasting

Following your faith's traditional days of fasting is a good way to not only overcome bodily desire, but to also look to the spirit life by focusing on prayer, meditation, or good works—it's easier if you worship in a community. (Avoid fasting if you are ill or on medication; pregnant, postnatal, or breastfeeding.)

340
Book an appointment

If you're over 40, then make an appointment to visit your doctor for a check to establish the health of your blood vessels, heart, and kidneys, and to discuss your diet and exercise and how to quit smoking.

341
Fiber fit

During a period of detox, aim to build your diet around fiber-rich foods—whole grains, pulses, fruits, and vegetables—to help your intestines process food and your colon eliminate toxins.

342
Cut out fast food

In a 2008 Swedish study, lean people who ate at least two fast-food meals a day, doubled their calorie intake, and remained sedentary, had similar

343
Steam treatment

The heat of the steam in this cleansing facial causes blood vessels in the skin to dilate, increasing blood flow in the area to promote the expulsion of waste products. (Avoid if you are pregnant or have asthma or respiratory problems.)

- 4 drops essential oil of chamomile or rose
- bowl of just-boiled water

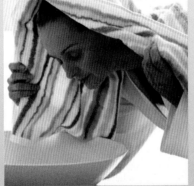
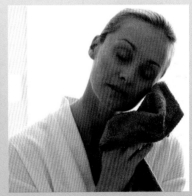

1 Carefully fill the bathroom sink with plenty of just-boiled water. Then add 4 drops of either essential oil of chamomile or rose.

2 With your face about 9½in (24cm) above the water, cover your head and the bowl with a towel to trap the steam. Breathe deeply.

3 Emerge after 5–10 minutes, and place a cool, wet facecloth over your face. Gently pat your face dry, then moisturize.

levels of liver enzymes after just one week to those observed in diseased livers. Apparently, it wasn't the fat in the food that caused the problem, but the sugar in the accompanying fizzy drinks.

344
Hold the salt

If you eat lots of processed foods, desire for salt may near the point of addiction, say homeopaths, and this can lead to chronic fluid imbalance in the tissues. If need be, try taking Nat. Mur. Tissue Salts for a month or so to reduce your craving.

345
Antioxidants

After a period of over-indulgence, a diet rich in antioxidants can feel

After over-indulgence detox with antioxidants found in green tea.

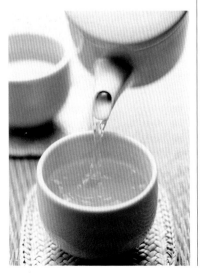

Dandelion is rich in antioxidant vitamins and is a great liver cleanser.

good: find them in brightly colored fruit and vegetables and green tea. Water-rich vegetables, such as melons and cucumbers, can feel especially cleansing.

346
Stimulate the thalamus

The thyroid gland at the front of the neck controls metabolism. Some yoga therapists believe that this exercise keeps it in good working order and use it as part of a daily warm-up: standing comfortably, point your chin toward the ceiling, bring your teeth together, then try to swallow seven times.

347
Cleansing breath

To cleanse your energy system, sit comfortably with your spine upright. Place your thumb and middle finger on either side of your nose just above the nostril but below the bone. Inhale through your right nostril and exhale through your left five times, using light pressure to close the nostrils alternately. Then inhale

through your left nostril and exhale through your right five times. Breathe easily and smoothly.

348
Tongue scraping

Many yogis and dentists use a tongue scraper when brushing their teeth, to remove bacteria and plaque from the tongue. Buy them online or in pharmacies or health-food shops.

349
Herbal support

A combination of *Chelidonium majus* (greater celandine), *Carduus marianus* (milk thistle), and *Taraxacum officionale* (dandelion) herbal tinctures makes a good all-around liver cleanser and tonic. Put 5 drops of each in water and drink morning and evening for a month.

350
Homeopathic remedies

The following symptoms are thought to indicate poor liver function; take the appropriate remedy once a day until symptoms improve:
• Lycopodium 30: if irritable on waking, plus gassy digestion, floating stools, or pain in right shoulder.
• Nux. Vom. 30: for constipation, cravings for stimulants such as coffee, and nasal congestion after alcohol.
• Sepia 30: for right-sided headaches, difficulty digesting milk, or PMS.

Sleep into shape

Since the second half of the 20th century, we've lost an average two hours' sleep a night, and people who don't sleep well may be more vulnerable to obesity, say a number of studies. Sleep deprivation may boost levels of the hormone leptin, which triggers feelings of being sated, and increase levels of ghrelin, which increases our taste for high-calorie foods. Here are ways to ensure you get the 7–9 hours' sleep most of us need.

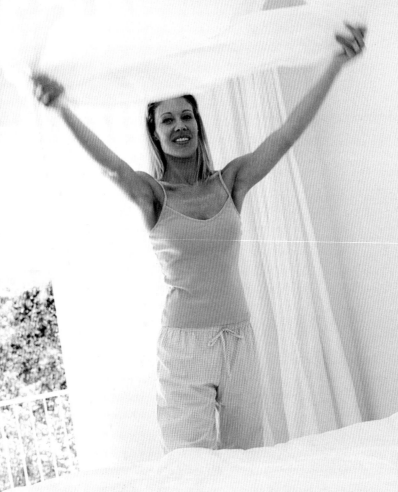

Aid sleep by freshening up your room—change the sheets and open a window.

351
Just chill

If your schedule means you can only exercise in the evening, you may be too hyped up or hot to sleep well. Try not to exercise within four hours of going to bed, or replace high-energy cardiovascular exercise, such as street dance or tennis, for a more meditative form, such as swimming or yoga.

352
Make a plan

Work out how you can manage a walk tomorrow and write it in your diary. In a study reported in the journal *Sleep*, people who walked more than six blocks a day at a brisk pace halved their sleep problems.

353
Refresh your room

Put on fresh sheets, relax the lighting (use side lights), and open a window to reduce stuffiness. Unplug all electronic equipment.

354
Eat early

Try shifting your main evening meal to before 7pm, and avoid alcohol and caffeine thereafter. If hungry later, eat calming carbs, such as rice cakes or a banana. They boost levels of the soporific amino acid tryptophan.

355
Shoulder balance

To rest your internal organs and aid sleep, lie on the floor with your buttocks 1 foot (30cm) away from a wall. Lift your legs up the wall.

Balance your body weight on your shoulders to rest your internal organs.

Bend your knees and lift your hips toward the ceiling; place your hands on the back of your waist, keeping your body weight on your elbows. Straighten your legs if you can. Breathe easily and comfortably in the pose. To come down, release your hands and slowly lower your hips—to tone your core muscles, bring down your pelvis last.

356
Relaxing routine

Establishing a bedtime routine lulls body and mind into a sleepy state. Turn off electronic entertainment early and quietly relax with your diary or a puzzle; have a milky drink and warm bath, then read in bed or listen to a story on your iPod before turning out the light at a set time.

357
Close shop

Close down your home as part of your bedtime routine: lock doors and turn off lights and electronic equipment; wash and dry the dishes and put them away. Such lulling activity serves as an act of closure and also curbs late-night snacking, which can increase your daily calorie intake significantly, found a University of Texas study.

358
Sleeping bath bag

These herbs and essential oils are renowned for their soporific properties. If you are going to be drinking alcohol or driving, omit the clary sage.

4 tbsp dried lavender flowers
4 tbsp dried chamomile flowers
3 drops essential oil of clary sage

Pile the herbs into the center of a square of muslin, drop on the essential oil, and tie to secure. Float in the tub while the bath runs.

359
Healthy hot chocolate

All you need to make delicious hot chocolate is cocoa, milk, and sugar, eliminating numerous ingredients found in low-fat hot chocolate mixes, from anti-caking agents to chemical flavorings.

1 mug low-fat milk
2 tsp cocoa
½ tsp muscovado (brown) sugar

Pour the milk into a pan and add the cocoa and sugar. Turn on the heat and whisk as it warms to dissolve the cocoa and add bubbles. **Pour into the mug** and enjoy while hot. Keep a teaspoon on hand to stir (cocoa can sink to the bottom).

360
Go to bed later

You may not sleep well because you go to bed too early. Try staying up until midnight—could you find a gently engrossing hobby to occupy the evening, such as doing crossword puzzles, beading or sewing?

361
Make time for sex

Sleepless nights may leave you too tired for it, but sex burns calories and the hormones it triggers can enhance sleep. Stop watching evening TV with your partner and go to bed instead once or twice a week.

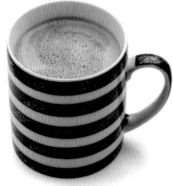

Make your own healthy hot chocolate using just cocoa, milk, and sugar.

362
Sexy flowers

Tiredness and stress lead to sexual apathy. These Bach Flower Essences may help. Place 4 drops in water and sip until symptoms subside.
• Olive: for worn-out caregivers, such as the mom who takes care of children all day and has nothing left to give her partner.
• Oak: for the strong but over-conscientious, who take on too much, leaving no energy for fun.

363
Drink up

Drink a glass of water before bed so you don't wake feeling dehydrated, especially if you drank alcohol during the evening.

364
Play with pillows

If you find it difficult to get comfortable, especially while

pregnant, experiment with pillows: place one beneath your knees if you sleep on your back and under your top thigh and knee if you sleep on your side. Try a lower or firmer pillow beneath your head for more restful neck alignment.

365
Count your breath

As you lie in bed, try to bat away worries by counting your breath. Count one on the in-breath and one on the out-breath, then two on the next in- and out-breaths and so on. Your mind might wander, but keep steering it back to the count.

366
Turn off your troubles

Keep a journal at your bedside to jot down concerns that keep you awake—such as tomorrow's schedule—then turn your thoughts away from them. If those thoughts shout for attention, imagine a volume button and turn it down—the thoughts are still there, but you don't have to listen to them.

367
Get up

If you're not drifting off, get up and do something, but keep it unstimulating: read a dull book, memorize a long poem, or pay your bills.

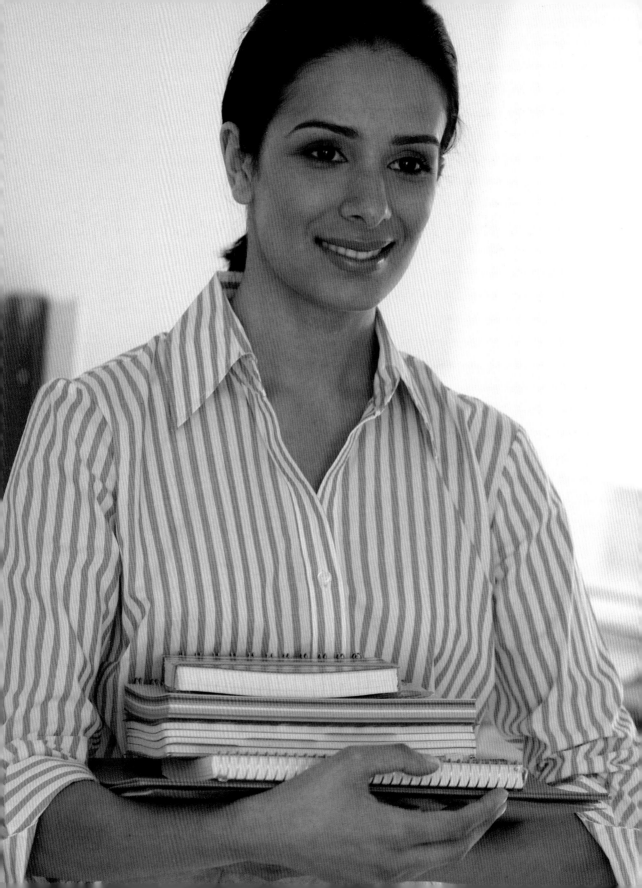

3 Workout in your work life

Americans tend to work longer hours and take shorter vacations than workers elsewhere in the world, such as in Europe and Japan—so if you don't keep up your shape-up resolutions in the workplace, you're unlikely to meet fitness or weight targets. Other research indicates that people who regularly work more than 48 hours a week tend to eat unhealthily and drink and smoke more than those who work more manageable hours. They are also have an increased risk of heart disease, diabetes, and stress-related illness. This chapter is filled with tips to help you cut your hours, where possible, fit in more healthy foods, and, above all, engage in more activity as a routine part of your working day.

Active at your desk

Studies have found that the average American adult spends 70 percent of the working day sitting. This can lead to postural problems, such as back pain, neck and shoulder problems, or difficulty in breathing deeply. Prolonged periods of sitting have also been linked to increased risk of blood clots. Here are some self-help solutions, from chairs that encourage active sitting to stretches and toning exercises you can do at your desk.

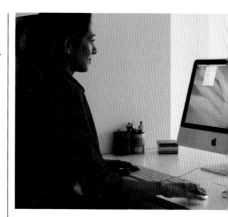

Correctly positioned arms and wrists will prevent upper body stress when typing.

368
Breathe out

Sitting at a desk encourages the shoulders to roll forward and the chest to bow inward. It's difficult to breathe out fully in this position. If you don't exhale enough, you don't effectively rid your body of toxins such as carbon dioxide, and can't take a full in-breath to energize your cells with oxygen. Every hour, stand up, roll your shoulders, breathe in, and then breathe out for a count of 4. Repeat the long out-breath 5 times, allowing fresh air to rush in after each one.

369
Counter cellulite

Some physical therapists attribute cellulite to long hours spent sitting on a chair, which puts pressure on the buttocks and lower thigh muscles, impeding blood flow. Stand up every hour and give your buttocks and thighs a good pounding with your fists, keeping your wrists loose (let them bounce off your skin).

370
Request a new chair

If the backrest and seat-height angle aren't adjustable on your current work chair, you need a new one. Talk to your boss or union representative about it.

371
New style chairs

Ergonomic chairs preserve the spine's natural S-shaped curve and position your body weight safely. Look for a saddle seat, which keeps the hip joints ideally aligned, a Swedish kneeling chair, or a neutral-position abdominal stool that angles your upper body forward and has a rest at your abdomen that reminds you to engage the core muscles that support your frame while you work.

372
Strap on a backrest

Favor backrests with an adjustable strap that you can move to the best position to support your lumbar spine (lower back). The vertebrae here support most of your body weight and are subject to most stress.

373
Rock and roll

Keep your back active on any chair by rocking from one buttock to the other. Then roll forward and back by pressing your sitting bones toward the back of the chair, then toward the front of the seat.

374
Check your desk

After fitting your chair to your frame (see No. 380), push your seat to your desk. Is your desk too high or too low? Could you reduce the length of the legs or place the legs on wooden blocks? (On a wooden table, you could screw a large wooden door knob to the bottom of each leg.)

375
Half stand up

A higher desk can counter a bad sitting posture. Raise your desk so it's half your height (the height of a breakfast bar). Choose a high chair or stool that allows your thighs to slope downward when your feet are flat on the floor (a supported standing position).

376
Use a footrest

If your feet don't reach comfortably to the floor, place them on a footrest or use old telephone books.

377
Keyboard etiquette

To avoid stressing your upper body, adjust your desk and chair so your wrists are lower than your elbows when you use a keyboard (your wrists should be flat when you type). Check that you aren't hunching your shoulders to achieve this.

378
Adjust your screen

Place your monitor directly in front of you, about an arm's distance or more away—turning to type risks injuring the neck or spine and reducing your range of movement.

379
Screen view

Move documents to the top of the screen so you look directly at them. Bending forward causes neck and shoulder tension. Increase the text size if necessary.

380
Adjust your chair

We all have differently curved backs and leg lengths; to keep your body working well and avoid injury, adjust your office chair to fit your frame.

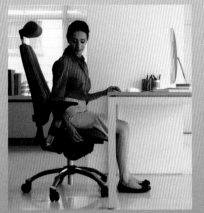 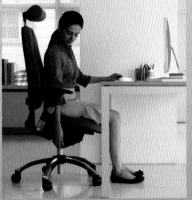 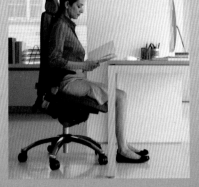

1 Adjust the height so that when you sit, your buttocks are at the back of the seat with thighs supported. Keep the soles of both feet flat on the floor.

2 Tilt the seat: the ideal position is a 110-degree angle between spine and legs. Check that your hips are level with or above your knees.

3 Adjust the back of the seat so it supports your lower back when you sit upright with ears over shoulders and shoulders over hips.

381
Active sitting

Spend short periods sitting on a large exercise ball at your desk. You could also make it your meeting or phone-call ball. When you slump or roll backward, it's time to get up.

382
Choosing an exercise ball

Make sure the soles of your feet are flat on the floor when you sit on an exercise ball. This encourages you to use the core muscles in your abdomen to support your spine and maintain balance.

383
Try a ball seat

An ergonomic chair with a seat formed by an exercise ball is better for long-term sitting than a ball on its own because it has a back support and legs fitted with casters for easy movement.

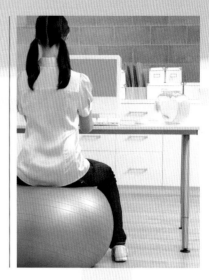

Keep a large exercise ball by your desk and use it to help maintain good posture.

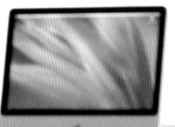

Tone your limbs by doing stretches using a Pilates band while sitting at your desk.

384
Exercise your neck

Sit up tall, widen your chest, and draw your shoulder blades toward your waist. Push your chin forward, then draw it in. Repeat the chin slide 5 times; imagine your chin gliding along a bar, keeping your ears level.

385
Boost foot circulation

If you tend to sit still at your desk for hours on end, wear shoes with tiny dimples on the footbed that stimulate pressure points on the soles of your feet. Pace your feet up and down as you work to increase circulation. Focus particularly on the middle of the arch where the venous plexus veins are—these pump blood back to your heart when compressed.

386
Take a band break

Keep a fitness/Pilates band in your desk drawer. To tone your legs, sit on a chair, place your foot in the band, holding one end in each hand, and stretch your leg out in front of you. Push hard into the band. To work your arms, hold the band with your hands a little wider apart than your shoulders. Raise your hands above your head and try to pull them apart; the band makes this challenging.

Snack while you work

If you eat breakfast before getting to work, you're insulated against unhealthy snacks. But as a second line of defense, keep some healthy snacks within reach, making it less likely that you'll trek out for an ice cream cone or a lunchtime pig-out. Keep enough snacks to pass around—it's easiest to change your eating habits if those around you join in too.

387
Set a time to snack

Try to resist nibbling your way through the working day, even if the snacks you eat are healthy. It's good to feel hungry before lunch and dinner. Instead, adopt set snack times, such as mid-morning and mid-afternoon.

388
An apple a day

Apples are one of the few fruits that are available almost year-round: keep one in your bag, changing variety with the seasons. One apple contains nearly a fifth of the fiber you need in a day and only around 80 calories. Keep the skin on for extra fiber if the fruit is organic.

389
Top snacks to stash

Keep these handy at work to stave off hunger pangs—they are filling because they are fiber-rich:

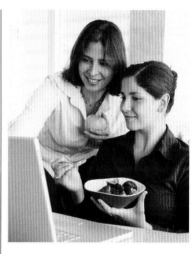

Fruit is the perfect workplace snack: apples and fresh berries will keep hunger at bay.

- Whole grain crackers
- Dried figs and dates
- Mini packs of currants or raisins
- Fresh raspberries and blackberries

390
A serving size

Each portion of fruit you have should be about the size of a tennis ball or a light bulb. Keep a snack bowl this size at work and fill it with berries, grapes, pineapple, or melon.

391
Big flavor foods

When food packs a flavor punch, you need to eat less of it. For example, 2–4 dice-sized cubes of Parmesan cheese, a few anchovy-stuffed olives, or squares of 70 percent cocoa-solid chocolate will assuage the munchies more effectively and leave you feeling more satisfied than processed snack foods such as tortilla chips.

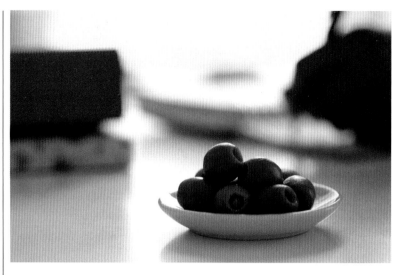

Eat foods big on flavor to help beat the munchies without the need for large quantities.

392
Mid-morning snack

If you're ravenous mid-morning because you skipped breakfast, go out for a filling snack, such as a whole wheat bagel topped with low-fat cream cheese and smoked salmon. Skip the butter; you won't notice if you ask for extra black pepper and lemon juice.

393
Snack on almonds

In a study of obese and overweight older people at the City of Hope National Medical Center in California, those who enriched their high-carb, low-calorie diet with 3oz (85g) of almonds daily experienced greater— and sustained—weight reduction over those who simply ate the high-carb, low-cal diet.

A filling mid-morning snack doesn't have to be bad for you— look for low-fat combinations.

394
Playful food

If you need something to occupy your fingers while you work—or perhaps you are giving up smoking and find you need something to fiddle with to keep your hands busy—opt for food that you have to pit, peel, and dispose of: try unpitted olives, fresh lychees, and thin-skinned oranges.

395
Change your habits

Swapping an espresso for your usual full-fat latte, an apple for two chocolate cookies, and sparkling water for your regular can of soda saves more than 400 calories a day. Stick to your new regime for seven days to near a target weight loss of 1lb (450g).

396
Low-fat yogurt

The calcium in yogurt may help the body break down fat, suggested a University of Tennessee study. It was found that people who ate yogurt three times a day while also cutting their daily calorie intake by 500 calories lost more weight and body fat over the 12-week study than those who just reduced their calories.

397
Just sniff it

The Smell and Taste Treatment and Research Foundation in Chicago found in one study that the more often volunteers sniffed an apple, banana, or peppermint, the less hungry they felt, and the more weight they lost.

398
Coffee watch

Beware of the extras lurking in the coffee shop: adding syrup, marshmallows, or sprinkles ramps up the number of calories in a cup of coffee. Switch to low-fat or skim milk (standard coffee is made with full-fat) and choose the smallest size available. If you feel you need extra coffee to wake you up in the morning, ask for an extra shot of espresso rather than a larger cup containing more calories.

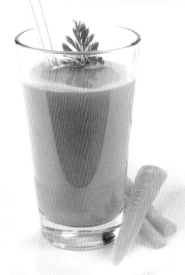

Kick start your working day with an awakening vegetable juice combination.

399
Have a cup of tea

Drinking black or green tea can boost your levels of free-radical-zapping antioxidants and can help to lower cholesterol levels, found an Israeli study; for greatest effect you need more than two cups a day.

400
Curb your hunger with milk

Lab studies show that milk-based drinks curb hunger pangs effectively, making people eat less at the next meal, while soft drinks work only on the body's thirst mechanism. This means that despite adding calories to your daily count, soft drinks don't make you feel less hungry, so you may reach for a snack as well. Instead, try a glass of chilled low-fat milk or a fruit milkshake.

401
Grab a juice

When passing the juice stall in the morning, grab an awakening vegetable juice: look for combinations of spinach, celery, carrots, and beet, or lettuce, with ginger for zing and apple for sweetness.

402
Afternoon treats

If you can't get through the afternoon without a sinful treat, make it a small one. To get a handle on portion size, measure your treat. In the US, muffins may weigh 5oz (142g) and contain 500 calories. A standard muffin 20 years ago weighed 1½oz (42g) and contained less than half those calories.

The size of a standard muffin is on the increase—consider the size of your treat.

Take a break

Many of us don't take regular breaks from work, although we know we should. But a culture that chains you to your desk for fear of being the first to leave isn't good for your health, your waistline, or your company's productivity. Research shows that people who work long hours become fatigued, which reduces their output and the quality of their work. Make sure you weave some breaks into your working day.

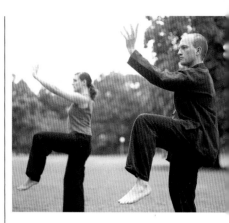

Be proactive: organize t'ai chi sessions and encourage colleagues to attend.

403
Know your entitlement
Research your state's meal and rest-break legislation, which should set out your legal entitlements. Look at the US Department of Labor's Occupational Safety & Health Administration site www.osha.gov and your state's labor sites.

404
Start working part-time
Join more than 25 million Americans who work part-time by talking to your employers about options to cut your hours. A 2008 survey found that 31 percent of US employers surveyed offered flextime arrangements and 39 percent allowed telecommuting.

405
Change workplace culture
Can you talk to the powers that be about starting an active employee program? Could they be willing to subsidize gym membership or loans for bicycles? Be proactive yourself; could you organize a teacher for t'ai chi sessions before work or lunchtime yoga?

406
Flexible working
Can you vary your hours or where you work to accommodate your fitness regime? Working parents who manage to achieve flexible schedules stay healthier than those chained to set hours, and have fewer episodes of physical and mental illness, found US research.

407
Use your brain
Switching from right- to left-brain activities every couple of hours helps you to take a break, deal with stress, and keep your mental faculties in shape. The left hemisphere governs activities to do with logic, calculation, numbers, analysis, and sequential thought; the right brain with intuition, creativity, and spatial perception. To switch on to the latter, try listening to a piece of music, practice yoga, or walk outdoors.

408
Set a timer
Set the alarm on your phone or computer to go off every 20–40 minutes. Walk around and stretch out to boost your activity levels and reduce the risk of stress-related health problems from repetitive strain injury to lower back pain.

409
Mouse break
To boost circulation and counter stress in wrists caused by too much mouse activity, stretch your arms in front of you. Try to grow your arms by stretching your fingertips away.

Raise your fingers to point at the ceiling, pressing through your wrists. Drop your fingers to face the floor and press through your wrists again. Now circle your hands five times outward. Make the biggest, slowest circles you can without moving your forearms. Repeat, circling inward.

410
Shake hands

Keeping your wrists flexed or extended (as in keyboard work) stresses the body and reduces the strength of your grip. Take a break every 20 minutes to bring your wrists back to neutral—the handshake position. Why not head around the office shaking hands to relax coworkers, too?

Take a break and climb the stairs so that you also boost your daily exercise quota.

411
Take ten

Every two hours, take a brisk walk about your workplace or around the block. Clock up the minutes this takes each time and record them in your exercise diary.

412
Use the stairs

When co-workers take a cigarette break, leave with them and spend 10 minutes walking up and down stairs (start slowly so you have the energy to keep it up). Do this even once a day and you could lose 10lb (4.5kg) over a year, states the US Centers for Disease Control.

413
Walking meditation

Try to switch off your brain for 15 minutes once a day by focusing on your breathing. Go for a quick walk; as you get into your stride, inhale for four paces and exhale for four. When this feels comfortable, see if you can hold in the in-breath for a count of two paces before exhaling for four. When thoughts occur, divert your attention back to your breathing.

414
Techno-free Friday

A Ball State University study found that use of phones, email, and Internet were substantially higher on Fridays than other days of the week. Could you ask your company to instigate Talking Fridays to force you to get off your behind and circulate among colleagues?

415
Take a lunch hour

A recent UK poll found that one in five workers never take a lunch break; of those who did, more than half took less than their 30-minute entitlement. If it helps, plan an activity, such as lunch with a friend, or simply sit outside for half an hour.

416
Feeling full?

The feeling of being sated is connected not only to volume of food, but also the number of times you chew and the amount of time you spend eating. Sitting in front of a screen to eat makes you more likely to eat your lunch quickly and swallow without chewing—people who do this tend to consume more before feeling full.

417
On the run

If you tend to eat on the run, try taking the Bach Flower Essence Impatiens. It helps you to slow down over meals and enjoy your food by giving it proper attention instead of rushing to the next objective.

Don't skip your lunchtime break—even if you only get outside for 30 minutes.

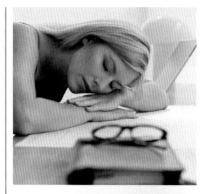

Improve afternoon productivity levels by taking a 20-minute post-lunch nap.

418
Have a snooze

Taking a nap after lunch improves alertness, energy levels, productivity, concentration, and memory function, suggests NASA research. It can also make a weight-loss campaign more effective, and keeps the heart in shape found a six-year Greek study. Take 10–20 minutes if you can.

419
Think family-friendly

Look for a job at companies with family-oriented working policies.

Fitting it in

To fit exercise into your day, you don't need to find extra time, just adapt your regular activities to make them more active. For example, try to spend at least 10 minutes of every hour moving around rather than sitting—even just standing burns three times as many calories per hour. And fidget, which may be as important in controlling weight gain as "real" exercise.

420
Spread your digits
To keep your feet and hands mobile while sitting at your desk, slip off your shoes, then make fists and scrunch up your toes. Slowly spread your fingers and toes for a count of five, trying to stretch your little fingers/toes as far as possible from your thumbs/big toes. It helps to look at your toes.

421
Ready for the weekend
If you like to garden on the weekend, you require strong hands, wrists, and forearms. Build up these muscles during the week by keeping a squeezy ball on your desk; give it 20 squeezes an hour with each hand.

422
Roll your feet
Bring in a foot roller or massage ball, take off your shoes, and roll your feet over the bumpy parts to stimulate the nerve endings in your soles. This is particularly good if you find you get cramps in your feet from sitting still for too long.

423
Stand up to work
Make phone calls standing up; on cordless, mobiles, and hands-free sets, walk around, lifting your knees while you talk.

424
Move around
To increase your exercise quotient, move around your workspace picking things up rather than asking others to get them for you. Be sure not to twist to pick items up. Position yourself in front of each one before bending so it's directly in front of you and within a comfortable arm's reach.

425
Offer to run errands
Does someone need a file, a ream of paper for the printer, something from the stockroom, or frozen yogurt on a hot afternoon? Become the helpful colleague who runs around for other people and get fitter in the process.

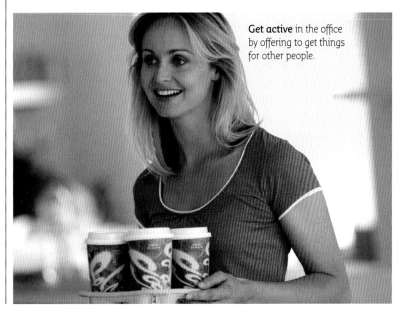

Get active in the office by offering to get things for other people.

426
Safe carrying

If you volunteer for extra lifting and carrying, do it safely. Stand in front of an object with feet hip-width apart. Draw in your abdominal muscles and bend your knees and at the hips as you descend. Hug the object to your body and place both palms beneath it. Stand up by contracting your abs and pushing into your heels.

427
Pacing with a purpose

Pace purposefully while you think, clasping your hands beside your buttocks and broadening your chest to increase the amount of air you breathe in and out. This increases circulation to your legs and at the same time helps to make you look like an intellectual!

428
Fidget

A study at the Mayo Clinic in Minnesota found that fidgeting was key to not putting on pounds if you eat well but don't exercise. Tap your feet as you work, flex and bend your fingers, fiddle with your hair. This is known as NEAT (Non-Exercise Activity Thermogenesis) and can help sustain weight loss. Increase your fidget level especially after over-eating (this really has been shown to work).

429
Thinking stance

To lengthen your spine and strengthen your quads while you ponder a problem, find a wall space and stand with your back to the wall. Walk your feet 1ft (30cm) forward and tuck your pelvis forward, flattening your lower back against the wall. Slide down, as if sitting on an imaginary chair, keeping your spine long and tummy muscles

430
Self-help reflexology

Use these simple hand massage exercises at your desk to relieve physical tension and raise energy to help you cope better with stress in the office.

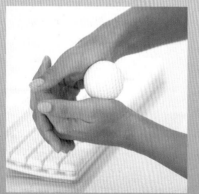

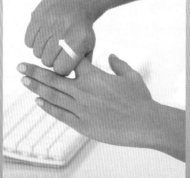

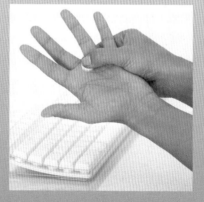

1 Interlace your fingers and place a golf ball between the heels of your hands. Roll it between both bases to stimulate the pancreas reflex point.

2 Make a loose fist with one hand, then squeeze and release the fingers and thumb of your opposite hand. Repeat on the other hand.

3 Finally, firmly pinch the webbing between your fingers between the thumb and index finger of your other hand. Repeat several times on both.

Hold informal meetings in a chairless space.

pulled up. If your knees veer beyond your ankles, move your feet further forward. Once down, take three breaths in and out. As you inhale, lift your arms up; as you exhale, bring them down.

431
Lost in thought
Use your body weight to strength-train your arms while waiting for a client. Stand an arm's length from a wall and position your feet hip-width apart. Place the palms of your hands on the wall at shoulder height. Breathing out, slowly bend your elbows to take your nose closer to the wall. Hold your nose just off the wall as you breathe in. Breathing out,

slowly push on your hands to return to the starting position. Repeat up to 15 times. Build up to 3 sets.

432
Project your voice
When giving a talk or contributing in meetings, pull your abdominal muscles toward your spine each time you exhale; this not only tones your abs, but adds weight and resonance to your voice.

433
Take your client with you
Can you plan a meeting at the gym or discuss strategy walking in the park? Take notes with a dictaphone.

434
Stand-up meetings
Arrange to meet colleagues for informal catch-ups in a chairless space—a hallway, the roof, the shop floor. When standing for a meeting, participants also tend to stick to the point and summarize rather than sliding into free-ranging discussion.

435
Throw a ball
For brainstorming, stand in a circle with a football or basketball. Throw it around randomly. Whoever catches it has to speak. This is a good way to encourage shy colleagues to contribute.

Lean lunchboxes

One of the best ways to ensure you keep to a daily calorie intake is to make your own work lunches. Food made and served outside the home tends to be much higher in salt, sugar, and saturated fat than home-cooked (or home-assembled) fare. Here are many alternatives to the boring sandwich.

436
The basics

When packing your lunch, aim to include vegetables and fruit, whole grains, and a source of dairy, fish, or poultry in each meal to make sure your nutrient intake is as adequate as your calorie intake.

Fill tortilla wraps with healthy, tasty foods for an easily transportable lunch.

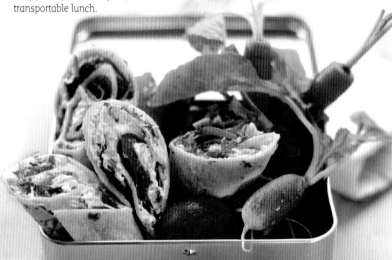

437
Pack a wrap

Wraps are good travel food because they are easily transportable and can enclose a variety of fillings. The following are good for keeping your bones dense (most of us don't get enough calcium daily):

- sardines, with chopped red peppers, scallions, and parsley.
- mozzarella cheese, with sliced tomatoes, avocado, and basil.
- goat cheese, with olives and shredded lettuce.

438
Paper wrapping

If you're concerned about hormone-disrupting chemicals in plastic wrap and sandwich bags, wrap homemade sandwiches in greaseproof paper or a brown paper bag. Avoid non-stick baking parchment, which is coated with silicon that can build up in the liver.

439
Hold the soda

A 2006 osteoporosis study found that older women who regularly drank cola tended to have a low bone-mineral density. To keep your bones in shape, accompany lunch with skim milk, Indian-style yogurt-based lassi, or calcium-enriched orange juice.

440
Bring a bottle

If you like something fizzy at lunch, take a large bottle of sparkling water to work. Soft carbonated drinks don't give you nutrients, but do add to your calorie intake. Carbonated water is calorie-free.

441
Moody lunchbox

To beat the blues and afternoon lethargy, make a chicken or turkey sandwich on whole grain bread containing sesame, sunflower, and pumpkin seeds. Add a banana, some dates, and a small container of low-fat yogurt to your lunch. All contain the mood-boosting amino acid tryptophan.

442
A handful of peanuts

Eating small amount of peanuts—around 20—at the beginning of a meal may help you eat less overall. Peanuts are also high in antioxidants and seem to boost levels of "good" HDL cholesterol and lower levels of "bad" LDL cholesterol. Choose unsalted, roasted nuts.

443
Avoid instant lunches

In a study of 21 ready-made meals at the Homerton Hospital Institute of Brain Chemistry and Human Nutrition, only two met nutritional standards. Sixteen were high in fats, most lacked essential fatty acids, and storing and reheating contributed to inadequate levels of antioxidant vitamin E. Their advice? Eat other foods—especially nuts, seeds, and grains—alongside ready-made meals to offset nutrient imbalance or deficit.

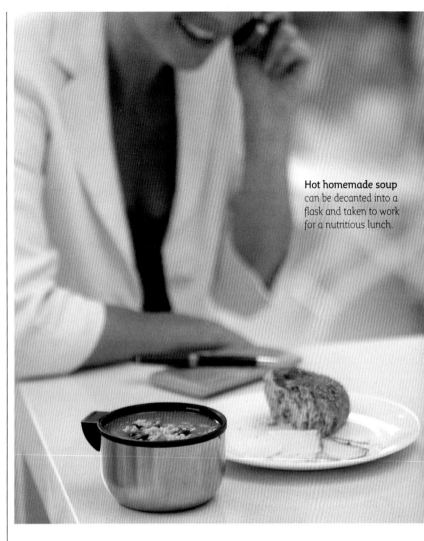

Hot homemade soup can be decanted into a flask and taken to work for a nutritious lunch.

444
Make soup

If you make your own soups, you can include plenty of vegetables and filling whole grains. Heat them up before work and pour into a wide-necked, warmed flask. Accompany with a chunk of crusty homemade bread and sprinkle a few shavings of a tasty hard cheese on top.

445
Portion controller

Measure out 1¼ cups of homemade soup and then pour it into a bowl. That's a reasonable portion for a single lunch. Pour that amount into your warmed flask for tomorrow's lunch, then decant similar-sized portions to freeze for future lunches.

446
Homemade minestrone
Make this the night before then warm in the microwave at work. ¼

2 tbsp olive oil
2 onions, sliced
1 leek, diced
2 carrots, diced
1 turnip, diced
2 bay leaves
2 quarts (2 liters) vegetable stock
½ cup cooked pinto beans
½ cup cooked green beans
1 ¼ cups pearl barley
2 celery sticks, chopped
4 leaves Savoy cabbage, shredded
sea salt and freshly ground black
     pepper, to season
1 tbsp chopped parsley, to garnish
shavings of Parmesan, to serve

Take lunch to work in a tiffin box, with each tin containing a different part of your meal.

Heat the oil in a large saucepan over low heat and cook the onion until soft and translucent. Add the leek, carrots, and turnip, and cook until they are heated through, then add the bay leaves, stock, cooked beans, and barley. Bring to a boil and simmer for 30 minutes or until the vegetables and barley are soft, adding the celery and cabbage 10 minutes before the end. Season to taste and serve with the fresh parsley and Parmesan. Serves 4–6.

447
Pack a tiffin box
An Indian staple, a tiffin box is a series of metal-lidded tins for taking lunch to work. They stack neatly with a carrying handle (which can slide onto the handlebars of a bike). If you don't want rice, curry, and dhal, fill one tin with pasta and sauce, one with salad, and another with a healthy dessert.

448
Cut back on meat
The average American consumes at least twice as many portions of meat as recommended, but not enough fruits and vegetables. And where America leads, the world follows. Can you turn this around by halving the meat quotient in your lunchtime sandwich and adding in twice as many vegetables?

449
Cut up vegetables
Take a pot of assorted cut-up raw vegetables to work to accompany soups and sandwiches: try carrots, celery, red peppers, snow peas, cucumber, and fennel.

450
Add fat
Keep mini bottles of extra-virgin olive or avocado oil and a wine or balsamic vinegar at work to drizzle over vegetables: your body needs some fat to help it absorb fat-soluble vitamins, minerals, and plant nutrients.

451
Spray fat
If you are calorie-counting, buy an olive oil spray that delivers one calorie per squirt.

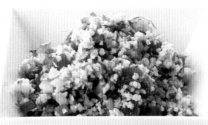

452
Take a tortilla
This is tastiest when cold; cut into thick slices to take to work wrapped in foil. Accompany with a few olives and a salad. (Makes 4–6 portions.)

4 large potatoes
¾ cup olive oil
1 medium onion, sliced
6 eggs
good pinch sea salt

Cut the potatoes into ¼in (60mm) slices, drop into a pan of water to rinse, then pat dry. Pour the oil into a large frying pan over medium-hot heat; when hot, add the potatoes and cook with the onion over low-medium heat for 15 minutes until the potatoes are cooked but firm (don't let them brown). Drain into a colander, reserving the oil.
Whisk the eggs with the salt in a large bowl and add the potato-onion mixture. Let it stand for 10 minutes.
Place 2 tablespoons of the reserved oil in a clean frying pan over a low-medium heat; when hot, pour in the egg mixture and whirl around so it floats free of the sides. Don't let it stick to the bottom.

Make a Lebanese tabbouleh using whatever ingredients you have in the fridge.

Cook until two-thirds cooked, 5–10 minutes maximum.
Place under a broiler to brown the top; don't cook until "dry"; the residual heat will cook it through.

453
Herby bean salad
This travels well—the longer it sits in the fragrant juices, the tastier it gets. Use ready-cooked beans.

1 can kidney beans
1 can pinto beans
1 can cannellini or lima beans
1 red pepper, diced
1 yellow pepper, diced
8 scallions, chopped
4 stalks celery, chopped
1 cup cherry tomatoes, halved
1 thick bunch fresh parsley
juice of 1 lemon
1 tbsp extra-virgin olive oil
salt and pepper, to season

Rinse all the beans, drain, and put them in a large bowl. Stir in the peppers, scallions, celery (add plenty of the green and leafy fronds), and halved tomatoes. Remove the parsley leaves from their stems, chop them finely, and stir in. Add enough lemon juice and olive oil to the salad to cover lightly, season, and toss. Serves 4–6.

454
Potluck tabbouleh
Vary this Lebanese salad to suit the ingredients you have in the fridge. Soak 1 cup fine-grained bulgar wheat in water for 10–15 minutes, or until soft. Drain through a sieve, pressing to extract as much water as possible. Place in a large bowl and stir in 3 tablespoons olive oil and the juice of two lemons, plus seasoning. After 1 hour, add finely chopped fresh parsley, mint, onion, tomatoes, and cucumber. Serves 4–6.

455
Picnic day
Once a week or once a month, organize a potluck picnic lunch with colleagues. The rule is that everyone has to bring something healthy—challenge participants to think of unusual picnic dishes and to bring them along for everyone else to try. For variety, you can spice up the event by suggesting themes, such as different types of cuisine, colors, or eras. Not only will this encourage healthy lunchtime habits, it is a fun way of getting members of the team together on a regular basis.

Eating out, eating well

America has one of the world's highest obesity rates; Americans allocate half their food-spend to meals outside the home. What's the connection? Portion sizes may now be two to five times larger than they were in the 1950s and 1960s—burger size has doubled since the 1980s, and restaurant pasta servings are five times larger. Research shows that regardless of appetite, we eat what's put in front of us wherever we live in the world.

456
Where do you eat?
In a three-year study, women who bought food in fast-food restaurants had a higher fat intake and gained 43 percent more weight than women who didn't eat fast foods. In addition, some take-out packaging makes it easy to stay slumped in a car instead of getting outdoors at lunchtime. Avoid fries served in a box that fits in a cup holder and super-sized soft drinks with funnel-shaped bottoms made to slot into regular-sized drink holders.

457
Fries don't count
In a Department of Agriculture study, when French fries were excluded from the daily vegetable intake of Americans, the average number of servings fell to below three a day. Remember that potatoes don't count as one of your five or more daily fruit and vegetable servings because they are considered a starchy food (like grains).

458
Soup rules
Clear broths—miso, minestrone, gazpacho—tend to have less calories than creamy soups. A study at Pennsylvania State University found that people who ate foods with a high water content, such as cucumbers (and tomatoes), ate fewer calories overall.

459
Walk to the restaurant
If you are eating out at lunchtime, choose a restaurant at least a 15-minute walk away from the office and resist the urge to take a cab.

460
Care for a drink?
If you tend to throw caution to the wind after a glass of wine—ordering more wine, extra side dishes, or the most indulgent dessert on the menu—could you make a rule to avoid alcohol when eating out?

461
Start with bread
Begin a restaurant meal with a little whole grain bread and you may eat less. Ask for olive oil for dipping. In studies, consuming unsaturated fat before a meal made diners feel full and eat less overall.

Eat a little bread at the start of a meal to curb your appetite.

462
Drink water
Drink a glass of water before ordering to quell hunger pangs and prevent you from over-ordering.

463
Salad bars
Any of these salad bar combinations are a good choice for a healthy working lunch:
- Multi-bean salads.
- Green leaves—the darker the better.
- Brightly colored ingredients—how many natural colors can you fit on your plate?

464
Hold the dressing
Some great salad choices come doused in high-calorie dressing. Instead, ask for mustard, lemon juice, oil, and vinegar, and mix your own.

465
Eat French
Order foods portioned up in France. One study by scientists from Philadelphia and the French CRNS agency found that portion sizes differed markedly between the US and Paris—French-packaged yogurt may be 82 percent smaller; a French soft drink more than 50 percent smaller.

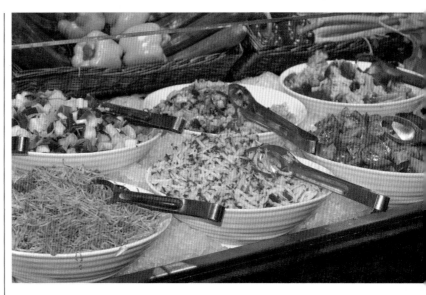

Opt for the bright colors of the salad bar for healthy lunchtime fare.

466
Eating ethnic
In America in particular, be extra wary in ethnic restaurants because portion sizes tend to be much larger than they would be if eaten in the food's country of origin. The American Institute of Cancer Research cites the Mexican quesadilla, which has doubled in size and calories on migrating north.

467
Unusual grains
Look out for unusual grains, such as spelt, quinoa, or amaranth, on the menu in restaurants when eating out at lunchtime. They are unlikely to have been processed. In studies, people who eat whole grains tend to keep off extra weight.

468
Easy peasy
What is the shapeliest way to eat out? Make sure vegetables cover at least a third of your plate.

469
Ask your waiter
"How big are the portions?" is a good question to ask if you are ordering plates to share, such as tapas, meze, or dim sum.

470
Half that portion please
Assess the size of sandwich-shop bread and fillings. Would you eat this much at home? Take a plate from home to gauge the size. Could you share with a friend?

471

What is the right size?

The US government publishes a handy guide to standard serving sizes for a range of foods on its Food Guide Pyramid. Visit www.health. gov/dietaryguidelines/dga2005.

472

Aides-mémoire

The British Dietetic Association gives these one-portion calculators:
• Cheese—the size of a small box of matches.

Portion size is key to eating healthily when dining out. Pay attention to what is on your plate.

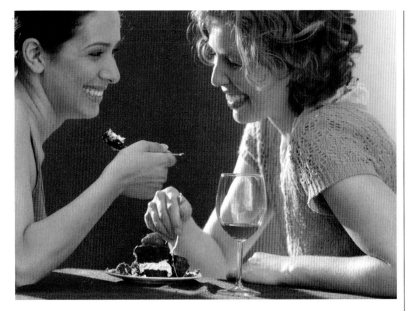

If you can't resist having a dessert, ask for two spoons and share the indulgence.

- Fruits and vegetables—the size of your fist.
- Carbs such as potatoes and rice—the size of a grapefruit.
- Meat—the size of a pack of cards.

473
Never supersize
A supersized meal from a fast-food joint—cheeseburger, fries, soda—could provide more than a day's calories in one meal if you are a woman trying to lose weight (1,500 calories). Could you switch to homemade lunches twice a week?

474
Eat all you can
Many of us do this at buffets, show studies. If you frequent places with a lunchtime buffet, use a small plate, don't go back for seconds, and limit yourself to one dessert.

475
Order fresh
Instead of helping yourself from a buffet, order from the menu. The food is likely to be fresher and you'll probably eat less.

476
Leave something behind
If you're known for clearing your plate (and other people's leftovers), try leaving one mouthful on your plate. Can you build this up over several weeks so that you stop eating when you feel full, not when the plate is empty?

477
Ask for small
In restaurants, make a point of asking for the smallest size of everything you choose—except salad and vegetables.

478
Share dessert
When eating out with a friend at lunchtime, if you find it impossible to resist dessert, ask for two spoons and share a single dish, thereby halving the number of calories you take on board.

479
Late ordering
Don't order dessert until after you've finished your main course. Can you really still fit it in or would an espresso do instead?

Do you really need a dessert—or would an espresso perhaps do instead?

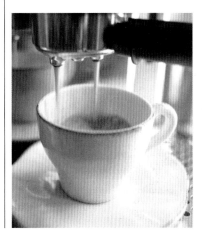

An active lunchtime

You can fit more than a day's minimum exercise quotient—30 minutes—into your lunch hour and still have time to eat. Then you don't have to worry about exercising for the rest of the day. Whether you get out to an exercise class, stroll briskly around the block, or walk to the salon, taking a proper lunch break reduces stress levels and increases lust for life, which helps you to maintain the motivation for getting in shape.

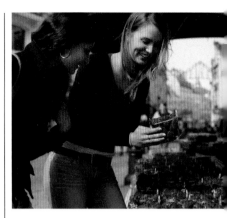

Take a lunchtime walk to the farmers' market and buy a healthy lunch or supper.

480
Step forth
A daily target of 10,000 steps is the equivalent of 60–90 minutes of moderate activity—more than enough to help you shed excess weight. Buy a pedometer and watch the steps mount up as you go window-shopping at lunchtime or walk to meet a friend for a chat.

481
Get outdoors
Spending time in natural light eases symptoms of depression in many people who get the winter blues (depression and obesity are linked in many studies).

482
Buy cross trainers
Lunchtime is a good time to purchase training shoes. If you're involved in a variety of sports, choose cross trainers that take you from jogging to exercise class to basketball court. Ask for advice on what to buy at a sports shop rather than a fashion emporium.

483
Sports soles
Slip shock-absorbing "orthoheel" sports insoles into your shoes or sneakers to make an active lunchtime walk or jog less stressful. These realign your posture and help to reduce knee and lower back pain by positioning the feet and ankles correctly—pounding city streets tends to cause the feet to roll inward and the arches to flatten.

484
Stroll the farmers' market
Do you need inspiration for a quick supper or for tomorrow's lunch? Walk to a farmers' market to pick up easy-to-assemble, nutritious foods: try cured meat and fish, local cheeses, olives and pickles, and artisan breads, as well as ripe local fruits and vegetables.

485
Walk to a flea market
Look for vintage breakfast bowls and dinner plates—often they're smaller than modern equivalents, helping to control portion sizes.

Buy cross trainers that you can wear for all your sporting activities.

486
Think thin

If you pass the bakery and your first thoughts are of the pleasure of biting into a pastry, look for your second thoughts. How will you feel if you indulge? Listen to this second voice—it is your thin self talking.

487
Stop holding your breath

If you are holding your breath after a stressful morning and have tummy ache, go outside and walk for relief. Breathe in for two paces and out for two paces. When this feels easy, increase the count to four.

488
Check out spas

Health spas suited to a lunchtime pop-in have quick-fix treatments on their menu, including sessions where two therapists work on you at once (perhaps on feet and face). To gauge whether a spa is geared up for a quick lunchtime turnaround, look for tell-tale words on the menu such as "results-focused" or "express."

489
Facial transformation

Get a lunchtime facial when your complexion looks gray or lifeless. Exfoliation removes dead skin cells;

Pop out for a lunchtime facial and return to the office looking and feeling rejuvenated.

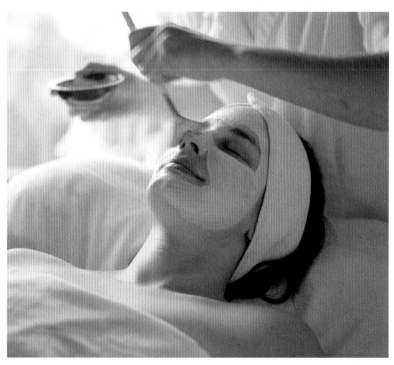

neck, shoulder, and scalp massage boosts circulation to bring nutrients and oxygen to the region and carry away waste products; while scented hydrating products lift your senses and replicate the waxy plumpness of youthful skin.

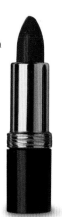

490
Splurge what you save

When you stop buying ready-made meals, fast-food lunches, or cigarettes, count the savings and put them toward a lunchtime treat—perhaps a pedicure, a new lipstick, or a DVD.

491
Leg rub

For afternoon rejuvenation, choose a pedicure that focuses more on leg and foot massage or reflexology than polish color.

492
Buy a new look

Does your usual weekly magazine celebrate unrealistic size-0 celebrities? Buy reading matter that celebrates more "realistic" women. Try these novels: Angela Carter's *Nights at the Circus*, Colette's *The Vagabond*, and Sylvia Townsend Warner's *Lolly Willowes* for inspiring fictional role models.

Fit a class at a swim stroke clinic into your lunchtime and boost activity levels while improving technique.

493
Get a haircut

For a quick fix to make you look in shape, get a lunchtime haircut. A good haircut can change the shape of your face and leave you feeling confident enough to relax scrunched shoulders, lift your head, and open your chest. This adds instant inches to your height and smoothes out the bulges.

494
Get a massage

In a study reported in the *International Journal for Neuroscience*, adults who were massaged showed enhanced alertness, completed math problems in less time with fewer errors, and reported lower levels of job stress. What better reason is there to book a weekly lunchtime massage?

495
Try an oxygen facial

Those who enjoy oxygen facials on a regular basis claim that this high-pressure blast of air delivering nutrition-rich products to the face firms, lifts, and rejuvenates tired-looking skin like no other treatment.

496
Shake your body

Vibration plates exercise your muscles at speed without making you sweat—you don't even need to change out of your work clothes. Simply step on, adopt the recommended pose (lunge, squat, crunch), and condense a one-hour whole-body workout into 10–25 minutes. They claim to burn calories, boost muscle strength, and increase bone density, circulation, flexibility, and lymph flow.

497
Sweat-free reshaping

Visit a flotation tank and experience letting go on a level you hitherto assumed impossible. Flotation induces a meditative mental state while allowing your body to release chronic postural tension.

498
Meet an Alexander teacher

A teacher of the Alexander Technique helps you to unlearn habitual patterns of standing, sitting, and moving that contribute to stiffness and reduced mobility; they also help you learn to use your body with more freedom and efficiency. It can have a radical effect on the way you hold yourself and move. It's best to have one-to-one lessons with a teacher; book an introductory meeting at lunchtime.

499
Swim stroke school

Does a pool near your workplace offer a lunchtime swim-stroke clinic? Get one-to-one or small group troubleshooting to help you power through the water more efficiently, coordinate your stroke with your breath, and link your mind and natural rhythm to find your flow. These classes help whether you're a new swimmer, training for a triathlon, have a phobia of the deep end, or find length-swimming dull.

500
Affordable trainer

Get together with a group of colleagues to have a personal trainer put you through your paces at lunchtime. A survey by IDEA Fitness Association, the world's leading association for fitness professionals, found that up to 71 percent of trainers were happy to hold two-client sessions; 43 percent would work for small groups (of up to five). They also found that group training increased client motivation.

501
Lift weights

As we age, we need fewer calories to get fat. To burn more calories, increase your daily weight-bearing activity at lunchtime—walking, lifting, carrying—and add in some strength-training exercises (squats, push-ups, rowing) for 20 minutes three times a week to keep your muscle and bone mass dense—these also decline with the years.

502
Grow your lungs

Yoga practitioners teach that by expanding the amount of time you hold an inhalation, you maximize the transfer of oxygen into your bloodstream and gaseous toxins into your lungs ready to be expelled. This keeps every cell in better shape. Practice breath retention at the pool one lunchtime a week. Start at one end of the pool, take a deep breath in, hold your breath, then glide underwater as far as you can. Keep relaxed. How far can you travel before taking a breath? Monitor your progress over a couple of months.

Shape up your brain by learning a foreign language on your lunch break.

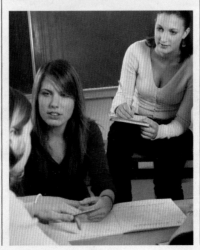

503
Active abs twist

To give your external oblique muscles a workout in the office, gym, or pool, stand with your arms stretched out at shoulder height. Imagine you have a broomstick between your wrists keeping your arms rigid. Look forward. Slowly twist from one side to the other, keeping your arms and face in line; build up speed gradually.

504
Health counseling

If you would like to change the way you live, but don't know where to start, talk to a homeopath. She will discuss your health and help you get an overview of your medical history and how you got to where you are now. She will then suggest remedies and lifestyle changes to raise your constitutional health toward its full potential.

505
Learn a language

A study at University College, London, found that learning a language shapes up your brain: like a muscle, the brain improves its performance if you flex it, building the area that processes information. If you're on your feet most of the day, can you relax at lunchtime sitting in a language lab or class?

Active afternoon brain

Our body clock ensures a natural energy dip in the afternoon; if you didn't eat a healthy lunch, your blood-sugar levels will tumble at this time, too. To keep your brain functioning well, try some of these energy-enhancing mind and body exercises and some snacks that stabilize blood sugar.

506
Raise a plant

Spider plants and peace lilies not only detox your work station, but it has also been shown that people who work in offices with plants were 12 percent less stressed and 12 percent more productive.

507
Enjoy drinking

Drinking enough liquids during the day helps keep the brain active (and quenches the appetite). Aim for 6–8 glasses of water. Make them more appetizing by adding a squeeze of lemon or a few chunks of cucumber.

508
What's in your water?

Before buying a bottle of water, check the label for sweeteners or even salt. Fruit-flavored waters may contain both. Tap water saves money and is greener.

509
Chill out

Chilled low-fat milk is a nutritious alternative to water.

Detox your work station with a peace lily, and lower stress levels at the same time.

510
Brew up

Commercial fruit teas may contain flavorings or sweeteners. Brew your own from plants that you grow on your windowsill at work, or keep fresh herbs in a glass of water. Add one of the following to a warmed teapot, pour over 1-2 cups of just-boiled water, and steep for 5 minutes before straining; add lemon juice or honey to taste:

- 1 tbsp fresh lemon verbena leaves
- 1 tbsp fresh mint leaves
- 3 slices of fresh ginger
- 2 cloves
- 1 tbsp fresh rosemary

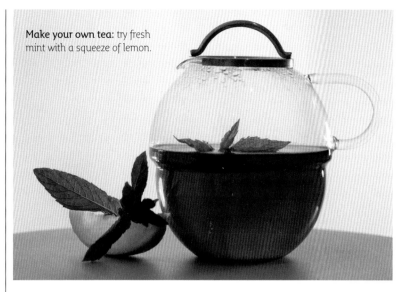

Make your own tea: try fresh mint with a squeeze of lemon.

511
Supergreen
Many users report that a supergreen food supplement based on algae, seaweeds, and other phyto (plant) nutrients helps to stabilize yo-yoing blood sugar and the resulting energy and mood swings. Stir the powder into freshly squeezed fruit juice according to package instructions.

512
Sprout seeds
Sprouted seeds are considered particularly vitalizing because they contain all the energy a seed needs to grow into a plant. Sprout them on a shady windowsill, then cut into wraps and salads or add to low-fat soft cheese on flatbread. Try peppery radish or mustard seeds or spicy lentils to pep you up, or nutty alfalfa, the easiest to sprout.

513
Dark chocolate
Keep a bar of 70 percent cocoa-solid chocolate in your desk. This will pick you up psychologically and also keep your heart in shape with its antioxidant flavonols.

514
Better cookie jar
High-sugar cookies cause blood-sugar levels to spike, then slump, leading to depleted energy, inability to focus, and irritability. Choose cookies made from oats, which release energy slowly; and nuts and sesame or pumpkin seeds, which contain mood-boosting fats.

515
Energy balls
One evening a week, throw a handful each of macadamia nuts, dried cranberries, figs, a sunflower/sesame/pumpkin seed mix, and dried unsulphured apricots into a blender and process. Form into small balls and refrigerate. Take two to work for a mid-afternoon fix of the complete range of amino acids.

516
Eye recharge
Lie on your back with your knees bent, close your eyes, and rest the heels of your hands on your cheekbones so your palms cover your eyes. Look into the darkness. Can you see how expansive your mind is?

517
Read a poem
To revive a flagging brain, change focus by Googling a short poem to read in your afternoon break: put woes into perspective with a war poem such as Wilfred Owen's *The Send-off*; when surrounded by a gray city try Gerard Manley Hopkins' *Pied Beauty*; for thoughts on time passing try Shakespeare's *Sonnet LX*, *"Like as waves…."*

518
Iron for energy

Iron keeps the hemoglobin in your blood distributing oxygen to all of your cells, and a lack leaves you feeling tired. Substantial numbers of women and young girls are iron-deficient, according to the US government. To increase your iron intake, snack on pumpkin seeds after a lunch of pulses, spinach, seafood, or red meat, and on foods rich in vitamin C, such as red pepper, kiwi, and oranges, which maximize iron absorption.

519
Think back to lunch

If you habitually experience an energy crash after lunch, it may be that you have some kind of food intolerance—wheat is the usual suspect. See if you feel any less lethargic when you substitute a rice salad or a baked potato for your regular sandwich.

520
Eat red

Red fruit and vegetables—tomatoes, cranberries, cherries, radishes, red peppers—contain plant chemicals that can help to boost your memory (and the health of your heart and urinary tract). Keep some in a bowl on your desk for healthy snacking.

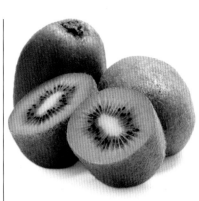

Kiwi fruit are rich in vitamin C—eat to boost iron absorption and energy levels.

521
Light up

You'll feel more active in the afternoon if you're bathed in natural light, especially if you suffer from seasonal affective disorder, so pull up blinds, draw back curtains, and clear clutter away from windows.

522
Revive your eyes

If your eyes feel tired in the afternoon after hours spent staring at a screen, book an appointment with an optician to have your eyes tested. By making close work feel more comfortable for your eyes, glasses can ease afternoon tiredness.

523
Simple leg raises

To energize the core muscles in your abdomen, stand with your feet together, draw the muscles around your pelvis and navel toward your spine. Point your right foot and lift your straight leg as high as you can. Repeat 3 times; then repeat on the other side.

524
Rev up

Place 4 drops of essential oil of peppermint on a handkerchief and sniff to keep up your performance at work and before exercise.

525
Energy boost

Ayurvedic practitioners teach that parts of the body that are closed in—toes and fingers, underarms, backs of knees—can act as energy sinks. When your energy and brainpower flag, stand up, remove your shoes, and spread your fingers and toes; raise your arms overhead and feel a stretch through your armpits. Flex one foot, then the other to feel a stretch at the back of your knee.

526
Full body breath

Stand with your feet apart and knees soft. Focus on your breathing. On an inhalation, raise your arms. As you exhale, bend forward and place your palms on the ground (bending your knees). Inhaling, imagine picking up something precious, then stand up and bring your hands to your heart.

Exhaling, give the gift to the world by pushing your hands away in front of you. Inhaling, lift your arms high again, and exhaling let them float back to your sides. Repeat until the movements become a gentle meditative flow.

527
Plan an activity

To maintain fitness goals, make a long-term commitment by enrolling your work team on a charity fun-run. Make it an afternoon activity to hassle participants about their sponsors and to plan team training.

528
Avoid confrontation

If you want to keep up diet or fitness resolutions, try to stay on an even keel when faced with co-workers' and bosses' idiosyncrasies, which may seem more pronounced when energy flags in the afternoon. Confrontation can be responsible for weakening of resolve.

529
Spray the room

Lift a dull atmosphere in your workspace with a homeopath-mixed flower essence room spray. Try Ainsworths Homeopathic Pharmacy's Cleanse & Protect or Ground & Go, which can be delivered worldwide from www.ainsworths.com.

530
Doodle

Get into the habit of doodling stick figures to keep up fitness intentions. Annotate parts of your body you like in blue and those you would like to change in red and state why. Over the months watch how the annotations change in color.

531
Neck and shoulder stretch

We tend to store tension in the neck and shoulders, which can contribute to stress headaches and hamper clear thinking.

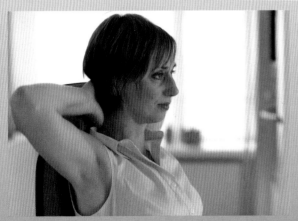

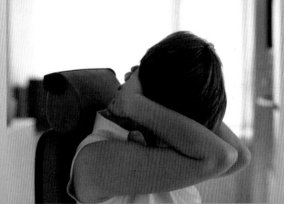

1 Sit upright and clasp your fingers together behind your neck, elbows level with your ears. Breathing in, press your elbows back, feeling your shoulder blades come together. Press your head against your hands.

2 Exhaling, bring the tips of your elbows forward and toward each other, dropping your chin toward your chest (don't pull on your neck). Feel your shoulder blades pulling apart. Repeat 3–5 times.

Energizing after work

It's all too easy to get into the routine of hitting a bar or restaurant with colleagues after hours or slumping onto the commuter train with a bagful of work, but this is a prime time of day to introduce some activity into your life. Exercise makes a good transition between work and home, infusing you with enough energy to cope with the evening's activities, from bathing the kids to tending to the garden.

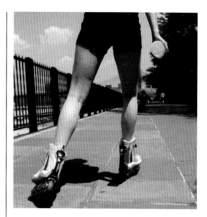

After work, learn how to rollerblade with colleagues as a team-building exercise.

532
Leaving on time
Are you a single woman in your 30s? A recent UK survey found that you're more likely to do unpaid work after-hours than any other group in the workforce. Start a discussion in the office about the reasons for this—and how you might counter it.

533
Working late
If your partner has to work late, meet near the office and go out for dinner to catch up with what's going on in each other's lives: couples who eat together eat more healthily.

534
Drink wine
If you like a glass of wine or beer after work, stick to one drink (two if you're a man). Moderate drinking offers protection against heart disease and stroke, diabetes and abdominal obesity. Consuming more raises your risk of cardiovascular problems and premature mortality.

535
Points planning
If you're following a dieting points plan, stick to core points-free foods all day and reserve your "treats" points for a glass of wine after work.

536
Alternatives to the bar
What else could you do to team-build? Try these options:
- Divide into two teams for bowling.
- Learn how to rollerblade.
- Try salsa dancing.
- Train for a half-marathon.
- Get lost in a maze at a garden open-evening.
- Be inspired by a contemporary dance performance.
- Book a guided nature walk or sundown birdwatching.
- Play mini-golf.

537
Start a team
Many cities host after-hours leagues for work-based baseball, softball, basketball, hockey, soccer, raquetball, and Frisbee teams. Send around an open email invitation to see if you can recruit a team. Or look on www.meetup.com for local teams to crash.

538
Slow runner seeks similar
Why not start a slow-running club for the truly unfit? Breather breaks are tolerated and sports gear disapproved of, but you must run for 10–20 minutes or more each week.

539
Women-only sessions
A Women's Resource Center poll found only 28 percent of women prefer a mixed gym. Women-only

spaces make us feel more confident, independent, and free to express ourselves—all vital for keeping to a fitness plan. Can you drag sister workers to a women-only gym or sports session?

540
Try cheerleading

Grab a bunch of girls from work and find an after-work cheerleading class in the gym or book a cheerleader to run a session for you. Laughs are guaranteed, making this great for mental health as well as toning up.

541
Try spinning

A spinning session offers the cardiovascular benefits of cycling with the camaraderie of a group activity. You sit on stationary cycles and engage in a virtual tour led by an instructor. After a gentle warm-up, you ride up hills and endure interval speed

trials and sprints. In an intense 30 minutes, you can burn up to 500 calories safely, as the exercise is low-impact and not weight-bearing.

542
Use a heart-rate monitor

These devices record your heart rate and allow you to up the intensity of your training to maximize aerobic endurance or take it down to reduce the risk of injury. Follow the instructions to establish your maximum and resting heart rates and training zones, then speed up or slow down your pace when running or in an exercise class accordingly.

Release the tensions of a busy day by playing Frisbee after work with members of your team.

543

Calm your mind

The IDEA Fitness Association, the world's leading association for health and fitness professionals, reports that mind–body forms of fitness such as yoga and Pilates keep people more committed than any other forms of exercise program.

544

Class etiquette

In a yoga or Pilates class, don't pull your legs or feet into position lazily with your hands—engage your brain and ask it to help you, then exhale and draw in the core muscles in your abdomen before moving into position.

545

Vary your workout

People who repeat a workout over and over tend to get bored and give up. Could you alternate jogging, biking, and yoga classes after work? By developing a wide range of muscle groups, cross training keeps you fitter than a single exercise form and also reduces the likelihood of injury.

546

Use the sauna

Studies suggest that a sauna offers some of the benefits of a vigorous exercise session for cardiovascular strength, blood pressure, and lung function—and burns as many calories as rowing or jogging. (Avoid if you have blood pressure or heart problems or are pregnant.)

547

Cold plunge

After the sauna, don't avoid the cold shower or plunge. It seems to boost

548

Active yoga sequence

To warm up in the gym after work, try this yoga sequence; it's best done on a sticky yoga mat. Persevere; it gets much easier with practice. When you start, it's fine to step rather than jump.

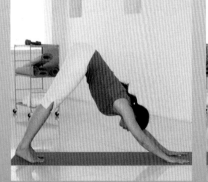

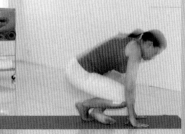

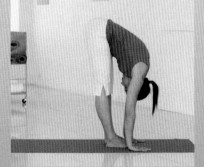

1 Inhaling, stand and raise your arms. Exhaling, place your palms by your feet. Inhaling, jump your feet back, hips up (Downward Dog). Exhale.

2 Inhaling, jump your buttocks between your palms, legs crossed. Exhaling, jump back into the Downward Dog pose.

3 Inhaling, jump your feet between your hands. Exhale your head to your shins. Inhaling, stand up, arms overhead. Exhaling, lower your arms.

immunity and blood circulation to the internal organs and reduce stress hormones. Athletes use immersion in cold water to promote recovery and performance.

549
Steam away stress

Try a *hammam*, or Turkish steam bath. After relaxing on a heated marble slab in a steamy eucalyptus-scented room to promote a purifying sweat, submit to a soapy scrubbing with a rough bath mitt followed by a pummeling massage to exfoliate and tone your skin. (Avoid if you are pregnant or have high blood pressure, vascular disease, or varicose veins.)

550
Get Rolfed

Rolfing is a form of hands-on soft-tissue manipulation, or massage, that aims to realign your body and change the way you stand and move. It can have spectacular effects on your posture and the way you breathe. Find a therapist for after-work sessions at www.rolf.org.

551
Thai massage

This is more yoga session than relaxing massage—a therapist uses her arms, legs, and feet to manipulate you into yoga-style

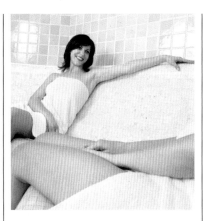

The heat of a sauna eases stiff muscles after a day at work, improving your mobility.

poses, and then massages you with her hands and feet. It leaves you buzzing with vitality.

552
Late-night opening

Many galleries and museums open during summer evenings or host recitals and festivals in their grounds. Distracted by art or artifacts, you can walk for miles and not notice you're on your feet.

553
Join a choir

Studies show that choral singing boosts positivity, alertness, well-being, and energy, increases self-esteem, and reduces the blues. In one study, a choral group with an average age of 80 had fewer visits to the doctor, eyesight problems, cases of depression, need for medication, or injuries—singing got them in

shape! In another study, levels of immunoglobulin A and cortisol were higher after participants sang Mozart's *Requiem*, revealing improved immunity.

554
Start a book group

Reading as a group may promote physical and mental well-being: people in book groups seem to gain relief from symptoms of depression and enjoy increased self-confidence. Or ask your doctor or counselor about useful self-help books; there is good evidence that they can support people with emotional difficulties.

555
Community garden

On long summer nights, there's plenty of time after work to get to the community garden. Look out for open evenings when you can taste produce and pick the brains of current owners. See CSA's website (www.localharvest.org/csa/) to connect with local farmers.

556
Learn to grow

Look for evening courses in growing vegetables or organic gardening. You might like to combine this with a seasonal cooking course on another night of the week.

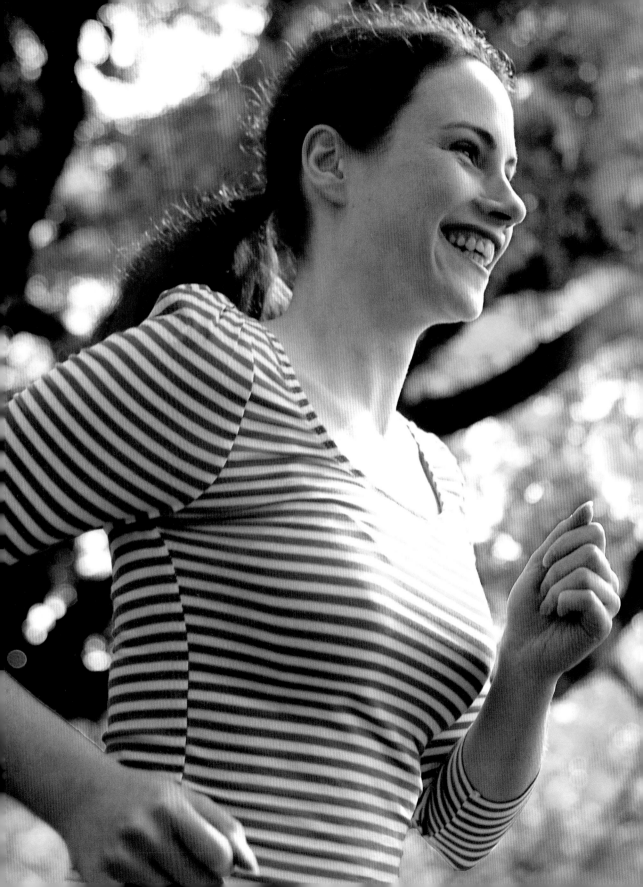

4 Active and outdoors

Average commuter times are rising, as are the hours we spend ferrying children to and from daycare, school, and clubs. The US Census Bureau has found that people spend an average of 100 hours a year commuting to work, which is longer than the average two-week vacation. One answer to the health issues this raises—from air pollution to rising levels of obesity caused by inactivity—is to shift your travel out of the car and onto your feet. When you self-power to work or school, there are no more unexpected hold-ups; being able to predict when you'll arrive leaves your mind and mood in better shape as well as your body better toned.

Get fit going to work

An average commute to work lasts between 45 and 60 minutes, found a Hewlett Packard study. If you let your body power some of that journey this is a great opportunity for a workout. Walking briskly for 45 minutes a day (about three miles) burns around 300 calories, which is enough to defeat fat and lose weight, according to a Duke University study; just 30 minutes' walking can prevent weight gain if your life is predominantly sedentary.

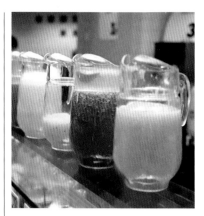

Plan your route to work to take you past healthy food outlets such as a juice bar.

557
Measure your journey
The Institute for European Environmental Policy reports that 38 percent of journeys of less than two miles are made by car. Measure your journey to work then see if you can you turn to a more active form of transport—your legs or a bike—to cover that distance. It takes only about 10 minutes to cycle two miles (over flat ground) and about 30 minutes to walk.

558
Workplace plan
Find out whether or not your employer has a workplace travel plan. They may be eligible for funding for bike parking racks, lockers, and showers, and trade prices for pool bikes. And you may be eligible for a mileage allowance, grant, or tax break to help you buy a bike under a bike-to-work or clean-air scheme.

559
Clear-head motivation
Biking or walking are a must if you often arrive at work with a headache and fuzzy brain or if you struggle to make decisions. Aerobic activity boosts "executive functioning."

560
Metabolism boost
Do you need more persuasion? Just 20 minutes of gentle cycling burns up to 100 calories. It also raises your metabolism, helping your body use food more efficiently and therefore maintain a desired weight.

Commuter breakfast: choose fruit over a pastry.

561
Find a free map
Almost everyone lives within a few miles of a bike route: look for routes and maps on www.mapmyride.com to plan your journey.

562
Route-planning
When cycling away from bike lanes, plan a route through traffic-calmed roads with speed bumps or quiet residential streets; use well-lit and well-used canal or riverside paths, but never footpaths.

563
Join a support group
Local cycling groups may be able to hook you up with an experienced cyclist who travels the same route as you. You can also try asking someone at a local bike shop for information.

564
Avoid temptation
If your new route takes you past a bakery, avert temptation by researching alternative routes—perhaps one passing a fruit stall or juice bar.

565
Eating on the run
Of those who eat breakfast in the US, almost a quarter do so away from home, found one study. But this is associated with increased risk of obesity because when ordering out, people tend to choose more calorie-rich, fatty foods than when eating at home. Break your commute for a quick breakfast, but instead of a doughnut or pastry, choose a grilled chicken sandwich or a peanut butter and banana bagel with some fresh fruit.

566
Thinking ahead
Before bed, lay out your walking shoes or cycling clothes ready to climb into the next morning. You're already halfway to your commuting workout without thinking about it.

567
Hide your keys
Make a pledge to walk or bike to work and ask someone to hide your car keys the night before you start to help make sure you keep your word.

568
Fusion transport
You don't have to power yourself all the way at first. Consider linked-up modes of travel, such as bus-walk or bike-train.

569
Get off early
To build stamina for walking, get off the bus one stop early each morning this week. Next week get off two stops early, the following week three stops, and so on.

Gradually build your stamina for walking to work by getting off the bus one stop earlier every week.

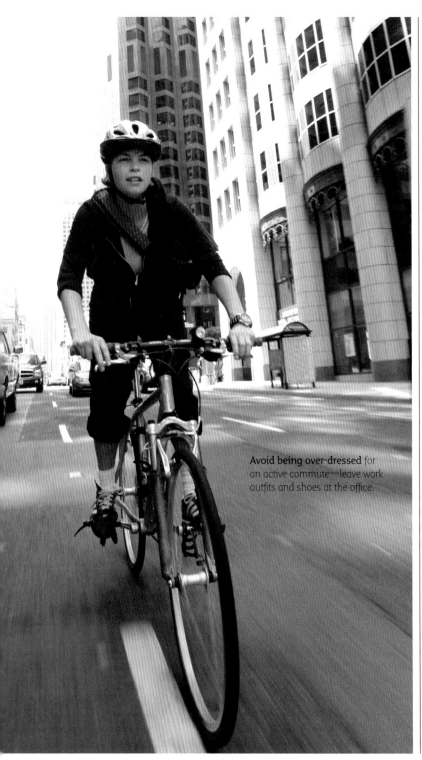

Avoid being over-dressed for an active commute—leave work outfits and shoes at the office.

570
Office outfits

Leave a couple of work outfits, including shoes, at the office (once they are dry-cleaned, leave them in the hanging bag). You can then actively commute without having to carry a change of clothes.

571
Commuting gear

Dress in layers for walking or biking, so you can remove garments as you heat up. You may need a vest, a T-shirt or base layer, a mid-layer fleece, and a rainy-day or wind-proof top layer. Don't forget a hat to protect against sun and rain.

572
Do I need new shoes?

If the tread on your walking shoes looks worn, you probably need new ones. Sneakers for a commuting walk should support hot feet swollen after 30 minutes of road walking as well as support cramp-prone cold feet. Ask for advice on width as well as length in a specialist sports store (see No. 607).

573
Take your socks

When trying on walking sneakers, take the socks you plan to wear with them and try them together.

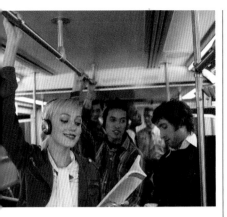

Standing up when commuting burns 70 calories more per hour than sitting down.

574
Get waterproofed

Owning a good waterproof jacket will prevent wet weather from denting your motivation. Lightweight jackets that pack away easily are good when space in work bags is at a premium. Look for features such as a roll-away hood, storm flaps, underarm zipped air vents, and a zip-in fleece layer for chillier days. If you can bear waterproof pants, choose those with easy-access zips that can be put on over boots or bulky sneakers.

575
Forward planning

If you don't have a fold-up bike (these travel unrestricted on many train services), reserve a place for your bike on a commuter train ahead of time. This will help to boost your motivation.

576
Memorize exits

Work out which train car is the farthest from the exit at your stop, then get in it daily so you have to walk the length of the platform when you arrive at your destination. Repeat on your way home.

577
Stand up

Can't get a seat on the train or bus? Give thanks! Standing burns 70 calories more per hour than sitting.

578
Core stability

To tone your core abdominal and spinal muscles and hone your balance, practice standing on a train or bus without holding on. Stand tall, with feet facing forward and hip-width apart, knees slightly bent, and ears, shoulders, hips, and knees aligned. Lift up from hips to underarms. Think loose and see if you can ride jolts like a surfer.

579
Get up and go with gadgets

Are you motivated by gadgets? Invest in one to encourage you to get up and go by foot or pedal power in the morning. Do a web search for heart-rate sensors that fit in your shoe and pedometers that talk to you, iPods implanted into sportswear, and hi-tech sports fabrics.

580
Striding out

Some pedometers come with a built-in radio as well as ways of tracking your number of steps and total miles traveled. Choose one that allows you to set your stride length for accuracy.

581
Switch on with music

San Diego State University researchers discovered that people new to exercise found it easier if they listened to music or chatted with a friend as they worked out. Think the same when you start a more active commute.

Make walking to work easier by listening to music on an iPod as you stride.

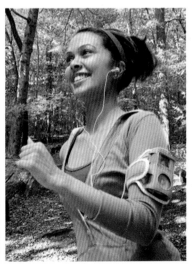

Active driving

If you do have to drive, postural adjustments can make it safer for your back, neck, and shoulders, helping you avoid injury and retain a full range of movement for longer. When you get to your destination, get active right away by stretching out, and boost your circulation with a brisk walk.

582
Car seats for adults
Ergonomic car seats lift you out of a slumped position and angle your hips correctly so that your buttocks are higher than your thighs.

583
Adjust your seat
Make sure the back of your buttocks are pushed up against the seat back so the whole of the back of your thighs are supported by the seat.

584
Empty your pockets
To help you sit up straight with your pelvis balanced equally on both sides (preventing lower back pain), remove everything from your back pockets, such as keys and wallet.

585
Driving stretch
To build strength in your abdominal muscles and those that support your

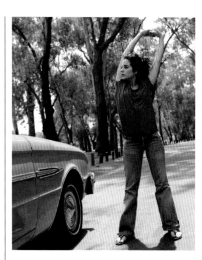

Take a break: on longer journeys stop regularly and walk, stretch, and shake.

spine, sit up tall, lifting from your waist to your underarms. As you exhale, contract your pelvic and abdominal muscles, pulling them up toward your lower back. Hold for 30 seconds. Relax. Repeat 2–3 times.

586
Wake and shake
Try to stop every 40 minutes. Walk around and stretch, then let your body go loose and shake everything out for 15 seconds.

587
Arm wrap
Stand with feet hip-width apart and arms hanging by your side. Pull your abdominal muscles toward your back, then swing your arms loosely so they wrap around your body; let your torso follow into the twist, moving your head to follow your arms. Repeat for 2–3 minutes, building up a flowing motion.

588
Park far
Park as far from carpark exits as possible, building more activity into your day. You're more likely to get a space, too!

589
Celebrate car-free day
Once a year, ground your car for the day. On Car Free Day 2004 in Montreal, there was a 90 percent drop in atmospheric levels of nitrogen monoxide and a 100 percent reduction in carbon monoxide.

590
Drive, don't smoke
Close windows when sitting in traffic. When you breathe in carbon monoxide from exhaust fumes, it reduces the amount of oxygen your blood can deliver to your organs and tissues. So does smoking.

Getting to school

The number of children being driven to school is at an all-time high, with fewer than 15 percent of kids walking or biking. A two mile walk or bike to and from school would help counter childhood obesity worries, and would reduce levels of nitrogen dioxide, which is associated with acute respiratory disease in children.

591
Make your child's future
Teach your children that there are alternatives to traveling by car. They are then likely to be less car-dependent when they grow up.

593
Start once a week
Walking to school just one morning a week—or once every 2 weeks—is a great start. Don't beat yourself up if you can't manage more at first.

594
Walk with friends
Children who travel to school with friends seem more settled by the time they get there, found a study by First Group Student (who run school buses). Walking with friends eases the transition from home and parents to institution and peer group, which many find traumatic, and helps to forge useful friendships.

592
Walk for your lungs
Aerobic exercise—walking or biking until slightly breathless—safeguards the healthy functioning of your lungs. If at the same time it removes your car's exhaust fumes from a busy road, then it protects the lungs even more.

Children who don't depend on cars are more likely to be active adults.

595
Walk to School Week
Get your kids involved in coloring competitions, poster-making, and star-chart activities during your own Walk to School Week.

596
Fund-raising
Could you raise funds to buy a bike for a prize in a Bike-to-School campaign? Or ask a manufacturer to donate one and give a talk at school about the benefits of bicycling?

597
Park and walk
It is easier to find a space if you park a little distance away from school. Gradually edge further away until your walk lasts 20 minutes each way.

598
Enlist the help of friends
If you live too far from school, can you drop your children with friends who live closer and always walk in?

599
Walking buses
Walking buses are simple but effective: adults accompany a group of children to and from school along a set route with agreed pick-up and set-down stops.

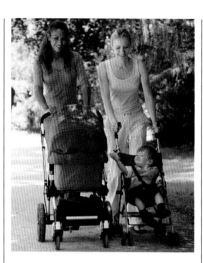

Walk with other parents after the school drop and catch up on their news as you go.

600
Adult eyes
Primary school children learn how to be safe pedestrians by walking with adults; they are then more likely to walk when they get older.

601
Discover nature
What can your child find on the way to school to put on a nature table: a fallen leaf, a pinecone, a feather? Raise their interest in the natural world while keeping them active.

602
Fruit alphabet
Liven up a boring walk with mind and memory games: ask each walker in turn to name a fruit or vegetable for each letter of the alphabet.

603
Walk and talk
Ask a group of parents to walk for 30 minutes after dropping children off at school. It's easy to sneak in extra activity while catching up on gossip.

604
Safety campaigner
If lack of crossing guards or pavements affect your decision not to walk to school, why not hold a public meeting to discuss issues with the police and local authority?

605
Choose a local school
Get involved with a school you can walk to. Become a volunteer or start an after-school club to create change in an underachieving school.

Turn walking to school into a nature trail, making it educational as well as fun.

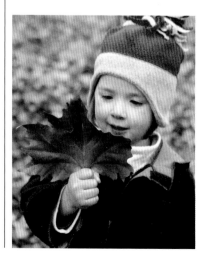

Walking tall

A brisk 30-minute walk—at a pace that leaves you slightly breathless—at least five days a week keeps your cognitive faculties in shape, eases stress, and raises energy levels as well as protects you from heart disease, stroke, diabetes, and many forms of cancer. Jogging and running bring even more health benefits, so up your pace whenever you can.

Ergonomic shoes such as MBTs strengthen your walking muscles.

606
Take more steps
Walking 10,000 steps a day (about five miles) keeps you in shape, reducing body fat and boosting metabolism alongside all the health benefits. But the average person only takes about half this number of steps. To build your step-count up, try to take an extra 3,000 steps each day. Keep count with a pedometer.

607
Get the right shoes
Walking shoes need to be flexible enough for your foot to roll from heel to ball with each step. Get fitted in a specialist sports or running store or one that sells ergonomic shoes such as Masai Barefoot Technology® (MBT)—these strengthen muscles in the feet, leg, bottom, and spine as you walk, relieving muscular tension and improving posture. They also claim to have an anticellulite effect.

608
Moisture management
Good socks make all the difference between blisters and bounce. Look at the options available at walking stores or online, favoring natural fibers, such as cotton, hemp, and pure wool—these allow feet to breathe (and don't smell, like synthetic fabrics do).

609
Push off
With each step you take, push off from the ball of your foot and again with your toes to put extra spring in your pace.

610
Look ahead
Your walking posture improves if you focus your gaze about 20ft (6m) ahead. Looking down encourages you to round your shoulders and collapse your abdomen, which prevents you from breathing fully and effectively. As you walk, picture yourself gliding toward your focal point on an escalator.

611
Tummy in
Imagine being propelled forward from your solar-plexus region (below your ribcage). Pull your abdominal muscles toward your lower back as you exhale to keep this area active.

612
Shut your mouth
Close your mouth and breathe through your nose as you walk to allow the microscopic hairs in your nasal passages to filter out car-exhaust pollution, pollen, and airborne germs. If you find that you need to open your mouth to catch your breath, try taking the level of exertion down for a few paces until you catch your breath.

613

Get a sports bra fitted

Forget any misconceptions about all sports bras having jumbo-sized straps: a well-fitting sports bra will make walking and jogging infinitely more comfortable. Look for a fabric and cut that provide support without restricting your breathing or movement in your chest and upper back. Seek advice and get fitted at a specialist store.

614

Try Nordic walking

Using poles as you walk tones your upper body: not only those hard-to-target muscles at the backs of your arms, but the pectoral muscles at your chest and the muscles that support your spine. It also helps to release tension in your neck and shoulders. Nordic walking burns more energy than regular walking (using up an average 20 percent more calories than regular walking, around 400 an hour). The shock-absorbent poles also reduce the impact of walking on the hip and knee joints. It's best to try out the equipment and learn the technique with a teacher. To find a local group visit http://anwa.us/.

Nordic walking using poles is good for upper body toning.

615
Use your arms
Coordinate your arms with your opposite leg as you walk, bending them at a right angle at the elbow and tucking them into your sides.

616
Healing foot soak
Ease sprains, cramp, or bruising by adding 20 drops comfrey leaf tincture (*Symphytum officinale*) to warm water in a foot bath and soak tired feet. (Avoid on broken skin, during pregnancy, breastfeeding, and with children.)

Arnica helps prevent damage to muscles, tendons, and joints.

617
Homeopathic remedies
Avoid jogging injuries by taking homeopathic remedies before and after your session (as well as warming up and cooling down). A combination of *Arnica, Ruta & Rhus.tox* in 6c potency (provided by a homeopathic pharmacy) helps prevent damage to your muscles, tendons, and joints.

618
Calming rub
Homeopathic arnica cream is an essential in any walker's backpack for tired, bruised, or overused muscles. When you reach your destination, take off your shoes and socks and treat your feet to a foot bath (see No. 616), then pat your feet dry, and rub in the cream using long flowing strokes toward your heart. Arnica flowers grow at high altitudes and have long been valued by mountain climbers, who chew the leaves to prevent muscle strain and increase stamina.

619
Foot warm-up and cool-down
This yoga-inspired sequence of stretches gently mobilizes your feet, toes, ankles, and calf muscles before you start a walk, and effectively stretches out built-up tension after a walk or jogging session.

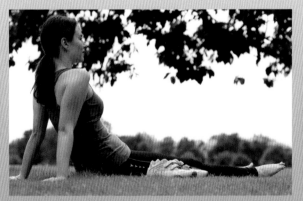

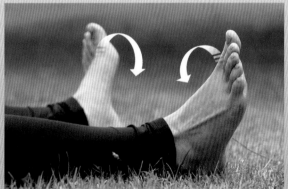

1 Sit with your legs out-stretched, feet hip-width apart, leaning back with hands behind you. Exhaling, stretch your feet and toes away from you; inhaling, pull your feet and toes toward you. Repeat slowly 10 times.

2 Keeping your legs outstretched, circle your feet toward each other 5 times. Then circle away from each other 5 times. Finally, circle both feet in the same direction—first clockwise and then counterclockwise.

Get on your bike

There's a cycling renaissance in cities around the world as people jump on their bikes, prompted by bike-hire schemes, bike lanes, and awareness of the environmental benefits of reduced air and noise pollution. Then there are the health benefits: regular cyclists have a fitness level of people 10 years their junior and live two years longer than non-cyclists. They also tend to have fabulously toned bottoms!

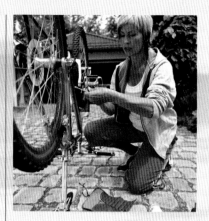

Keep your bike in good condition to ensure many miles of safe, trouble-free cycling.

620
Choosing a bike
It's important to get a bike that suits the geography of the region you ride in: is it hilly or flat; wet, dry, or salty; urban roads or muddy lanes? Seek the advice of an independent bike dealer. If you are still unsure, rent several bikes for an afternoon and get the feel of each.

621
Rails-to-trails
The RTC (Rails-to-Trails Conservancy) organization is working to create a nationwide network of public cycle trails by transforming former rail lines and linking up with cycle corridors. Visit their website to see if there's a trail near you (or to find out how to help build a new trail): www.railtrails.org

622
Get fitted
Adjust the height of your saddle and handlebars for an efficient and safe cycle workout. To use all your lower leg muscles effectively and stave off saddle-soreness, your leg should extend fully when your bottom is on the seat and heel on the pedal in the down position (which may feel unnaturally high). Adjust your handlebars once you're happy with the saddle height.

623
Cycle safely
Unless you know the life history of a helmet, buy a new one—and if you're involved in an accident, replace the helmet. Fit reflectors to bike wheels and pedals, and wear a reflective jacket, over-shoulder band, or backpack cover. Use lights at dusk and beyond, and fit a bell to warn pedestrians of your presence.

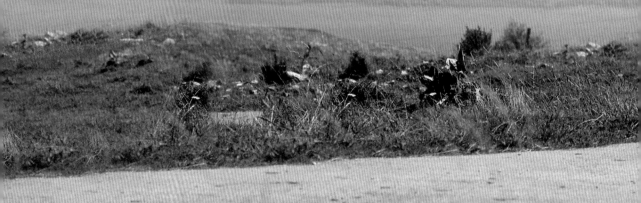

624
Clear ears
Don't wear your iPod when biking (unless you are on a stationary bike at the gym). You need all your senses to anticipate the movements of traffic and pedestrians.

625
Locking up
Instead of driving your children to the park, recreational center, or bowling alley, bike there with them. Make sure you can secure your bikes when you get there. Favor a D-lock over a cable lock, which can be easily cut off. You might also want to look into removable seats and pedals.

626
Starting again
If you haven't bicycled since childhood, practice on an off-road trail until you feel more confident, and contact the League of American Bicyclists (www.bikeleague.org) for information on how to boost your confidence and learn the rules of the road and basic maintenance skills.

627
Service essentials
Clean your bike regularly. Wash off mud, oil the chain, and check the tire pressure and brakes. Get your bike serviced annually by a CYTECH-qualified mechanic.

628
Carrying weight
If you're carrying work or shopping in a backpack or a front basket, be aware that the weight will affect your center of gravity and balance. Try to keep extra weight on the back and low: weight up front makes you wobbly.

629
Don't worry
Car drivers inhale more exhaust fumes than cyclists because they sit in a "tunnel of pollution"; at the side of the road, cyclists are exposed to fewer fumes, so don't let this fear keep you off the road.

When choosing a bike make sure you match the bike you buy to the terrain you are intending to ride on.

630
Own your space
Hugging the curb keeps you hidden and presents dangers when you need to overtake parked vehicles—bike at least 3ft (1m) from the curb. Use clear hand signals and make eye contact with other traffic and pedestrians.

631
Are you burning calories?
For every 0.6 miles (1 kilometer) of moderate cycling, you burn around 35 calories. You can use an online counter (www.caloriesperhour.com).

632
Keeping track
To track your improving fitness, follow a route three times a week for at least 30 minutes. At the end of each week, use a cycling computer to measure your speed over the ride. You should soon see an improvement in the figures.

633
Building fitness
As you get fitter, lengthen the route, adding 2–3 miles at a time, or add in more hill-climbs and sprinting.

634
Cycling for heart health
Cyclists tend to have a reduced risk of heart attacks and high blood pressure because cycling is an excellent cardiovascular conditioner. To really work heart and lungs, build up your sprint-cycling gradually over several weeks and months.

635
Exercising with a trailer
Pulling a child or a load in a bike trailer is a fantastic way to build muscle in the legs and heart.

636
Post-cycle stretch
This sequence eases out the front of your thighs, your hips and upper back, and the core muscles of your abdomen. In step one, step your front foot further forward if your knee moves beyond your ankle.

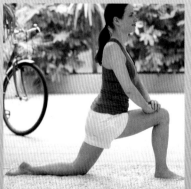 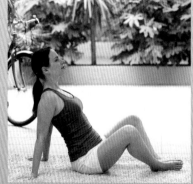 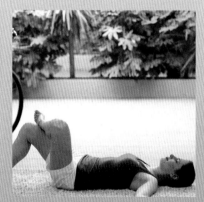

1 Kneel upright, step your right foot forward, place your hands above your knee, lunge forward. Hold until the muscle eases; repeat on the left leg.

2 Sit on the floor with the soles of your feet together, heels toward your groin. Place your hands behind you and lift your breastbone to the sky.

3 Lie on your back with knees bent, feet on the floor. Cross one knee over the other then drop the top knee toward the floor. Repeat on other leg.

Venturing further afield

In a 2007 study, two-thirds of vacationers questioned said that they put on weight on their trip—5 percent put on a whole 14lb (6kg). You may find that the reverse is the case if you take a vacation where you power some of the travel yourself!

637
Take your break
The World Tourism Organization has found that US workers take the least number of vacation days. This means you have fewer chances to get active. Exercise on the weekends to increase your opportunity for toning.

638
Biking for softies
You don't have to be a fitness maniac to enjoy a cycling vacation. Some are set up for softies: your luggage is transported from hotel to hotel as you leisurely make your way along scenic bike paths. Stop to explore an out-of-the-way town or take a leisurely lunch before riding it off on your way to your next eager chef, complementary massage, and soft bed.

639
Be your hero
If you are a cycling enthusiast, look for sport-cycling breaks that allow you to ride the routes of your heroes over mountain passes or compete in a time-trialed "raid," such as the legendary route over the Pyrenees from Mediterranean to Atlantic.

640
Use a map
If you tend to rely on satellite navigation when driving, head into the hills on a hike to develop the skill of map reading while boosting your fitness. Maps show points of interest from springs to nature reserves that you can trek to.

641
Charity trekking
A sponsored trek or ride for charity pushes you to your physical limits while building compassion, a sense of perspective, and self-confidence that enhances your regular life.

642
All-terrain training
Take a weekend training break before a major trek or hiking holiday so you can practice over a similar terrain and altitude to your vacation.

When out walking learn how to use a map to make sure you stay on track.

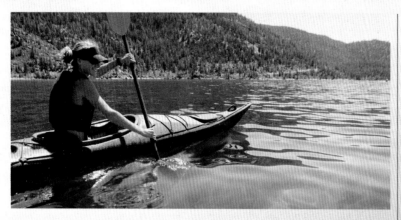

Kayaking takes you to places you can't reach otherwise, and gets you in shape on the way.

and dawn of a desert. Be prepared to walk part of the way to rest your inner thighs and buttocks.

648
Paddle there

Think of kayaking as hiking over water—getting you to places other forms of transport can't reach, from deserted islands to shallow-water

643
Gait analysis

Before a major trek, book a gait analysis in a sports shop. A technician will give an accurate picture of your "pronation"—the angle of your arch and the way your foot rolls and body weight is absorbed—and suggest shoes to rebalance your gait.

644
Trek-training

Even if you have an active life, train for your expedition activity for at least four months before setting off. Visit your doctor for a physical health check, then consult a fitness professional for advice on a fitness and nutrition build-up plan.

645
After-hike stretch

To stretch out your calves, hands, and arms, stand at arm's length

from a wall and stretch your arms above your head. Hold for a few breaths, then step one foot forward. Place your palms high on the wall and stretch into your back heel. Feel a stretch down your arms, armpits, and back leg. Change legs, then shake out.

646
Horse-riding getaway

Horse riding tones the buttocks, thighs, and calves, and strengthens your core abdominal muscles, since you learn to sit tall without a back support. It can burn more than 400 calories an hour.

647
Camel camping

A camel-camping safari is challenging for the thighs and buttocks, but also an eye-opening way to get up close to wildlife and the spectacular sunset, starlight, inlets. If you're not up on navigation, signaling, tides, and currents, or have never paddled a loaded boat, choose a guided trip.

649

Plan a pilgrimage

Walking is recognized as a means of spiritual awakening in the great faith traditions. A walk to a holy site or a place with spiritual meaning might take an afternoon or six weeks. Both are valuable: religious practices including prayer seem to correlate with reduced stress, lowered blood pressure, and increased health and life expectancy. The repetition and physical exertion of walking stills a chattering mind, which leads to increased mindfulness or a state of prayer.

650

Walk a labyrinth

Labyrinths are ancient symbols of the quest for spiritual growth. As you walk along the twisting path to a hidden center and then back out to the world, you journey to your own still center. Look for labyrinths at churches, cathedrals, and other spiritual sites.

Sitting tall: horse riding tones your muscles as well as your mind.

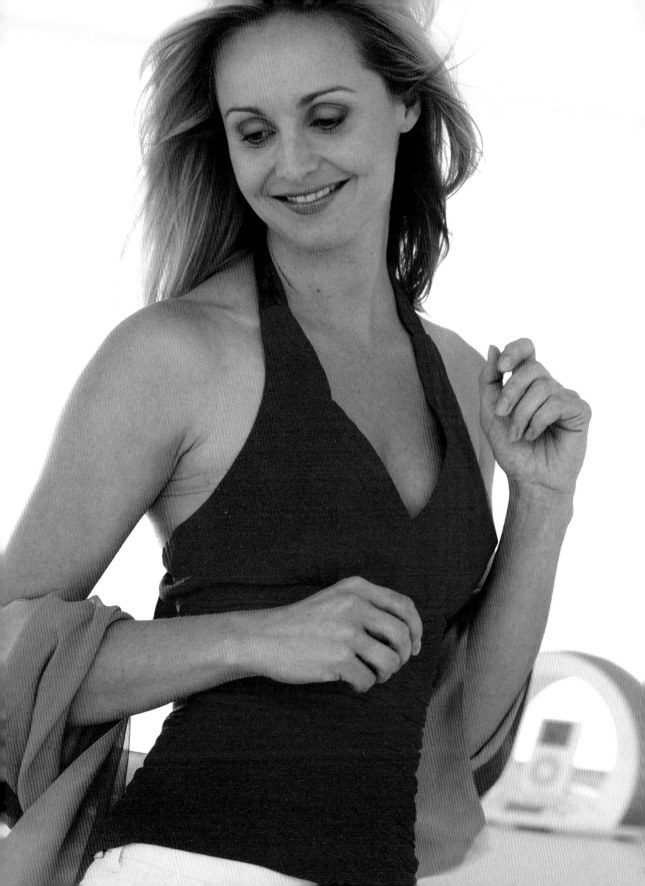

5
Have fun getting fit

Getting in shape isn't about stopping doing the things you love, it's about discovering fun new pastimes that get your body moving and activate your mind, and making time to fit them in. Playing not only hones your waistline, it keeps you in shape emotionally and mentally. Playing outdoors is particularly beneficial. Green exercise doesn't have to involve a wilderness experience requiring walking boots or a hard hat—any kind of physical activity that gets you into a natural setting (including small urban parks) counts, from walking a toddler to the local park to taking part in heritage projects to conserve the environment. But best of all, simply turning off the TV and heading into the open air is likely to keep you active for longer.

Turn off the TV

Television is still the piece of technology that keeps us most immobile. In the average home, a TV set is turned on for more than a third of the day—eight hours, 14 minutes—reports Nielsen Media Research. That's one hour longer than a decade ago. Most of that extra viewing is done outside of prime time, suggesting we're stuck on the sofa more often during the day.

651
Use your brain
People who keep their brains engaged with activities such as crosswords, sudoku, book groups, and learning new languages or skills, tend to keep their memory sharp and their cognitive functioning acute into old age. Turn off the TV tonight to start getting brain-fit.

Make the commercial break an exercise opportunity.

652
Knit while you watch
Watching TV lowers your metabolic rate. Knit or sketch while you watch to keep it up.

653
Switch off cable
The rise in digital channels has been mirrored by an increase in TV viewing, especially in older people, found a study in the UK. Can you reduce your cable package to a minimum number of channels?

654
Stop surfing
Ask your kids to hide the remote. Having to get up to switch channels makes TV viewing less attractive.

655
Yoga pose for TV viewing
Sit on a cushion with knees wide apart and feet in front of your groin, one heel in front of the other. Place cushions beneath your knees if they don't touch the ground. Keeping your knees slightly lower than your hips comforts your back.

656
Commercial break squats
Stand with your feet facing forward, hip-width apart, and imagine they are glued to the spot. Keeping your knees wide, bend them while you descend as low as you can.

657
Fitness Wii
With more than 40 fitness activities, the Wii Fit virtual fitness instructor demonstrates workouts to suit different family members, from aerobic conditioning to yoga poses and spot toning.

Healthy entertaining

If you're worried about taking rogue calories on board when socializing, invite guests to your home so you're in charge of the food, drinks, and activities—active game-play goes down surprisingly well at grown-up gatherings. Think carefully about the drinks you serve, too. Alcohol contains almost as many calories per gram as fat.

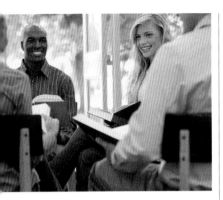

Keep your brain fit: turn off your TV and join a book group or learn a language.

658
Away games

Don't slouch on the sofa watching the big game. Head away from home to view sports events standing in a bar or socializing at a friend's place.

659
Sit on a ball

When viewing, sit on an exercise ball to stop you from slouching and to exercise your abdominal muscles and those supporting your lower back.

660
Radiation zapping

Televisions and computers emit radiation that natural therapists believe may drain your energy. Radiation Essence is a combination of Australian Bush Flower Essences formulated to counter the effects. Take a few drops to boost your energy supplies.

661
Walk before dinner

Take guests on a stroll before dinner; could you meet at a beautiful spot to watch a sunset before dining? In one study, obese women who took a 20-minute walk felt as full as if they had eaten a light meal.

662
Party themes

Build a party around an active theme, such as a baseball party, Olympic Games afternoon, or a woodland hike picnic.

663
Active party activities

Try these alternatives to sitting around eating and drinking:
- Treasure hunt
- Charades
- Twister
- Informal softball
- Frisbee
- Five-a-side soccer

664
Don't overeat at parties

Research suggests that if we eat in groups, we tend to eat more—the larger the group, the more we eat. Keep this in mind at parties.

665
Helpful host

Prevent guests from picking at parties by offering food only when it's time to eat and plate portions rather than inviting guests to help themselves.

Have fun playing Twister rather than just sitting and eating and drinking.

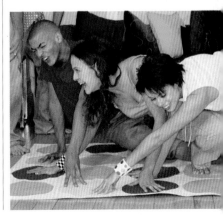

666
Circulate, circulate
To stop yourself from hogging the buffet table or bar, aim to talk to every person in the room.

667
Small plates
As hostess, put out smaller plates; when at a social gathering, choose the smallest-sized plate, or half fill a large plate with salad.

668
Let them drink tea
Make tea the new wine—green tea contains zero calories and is richer than red wine in antioxidant polyphenols. Serve in a beautiful Chinese teapot.

669
Iced tea
This goes down well at afternoon get-togethers. The sweetness of the apple juice replaces sugar.

4 Earl Grey tea bags
1½ cups cloudy apple juice
½ lemon, sliced
½ orange, sliced
1 apple, cored and sliced
handful fresh mint leaves

Place the tea bags in a large teapot and pour freshly boiled water overtop. Allow to steep for 20 minutes, then

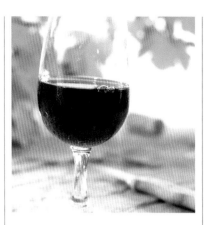

Avoid high-calorie cocktails in favor of a small glass of quality wine.

pour into a large glass jug. Let cool. Then add the apple juice, sliced fruit, mint leaves, and plenty of ice. Refrigerate and serve over ice.

670
Drink good wine
Alcopops tend to be higher in calories and additives than wine or beer. One 12fl oz (350ml) bottle contains just over 200 calories—a small glass of wine has around 80.

671
Alternate drinks
At parties, follow each alcoholic drink with a glass of calorie-free water.

672
Check the strength
Look at the strength of wines on a wine list. Choose one with the least amount of alcohol (and calories).

673
Measure your glasses
How big is your usual cocktail? Fill up your regular wine glass with water and measure it. Now measure out 4fl oz (125ml)—that's one unit.

674
Dilute it
Pour 4fl oz (125ml) chilled white wine into a large glass, then top off with sparkling water and ice to create a lower-calorie spritzer.

675
Look, no hands
At parties hold a glass of mineral water in one hand and wine in the other so you can't eat the chips.

676
Choose cooler wines
The hotter a vineyard's climate, the more likely the wine is to be heavy in alcohol and calories. For lighter wines, look to grapes grown in cool-climate vineyards, such as white German Riesling.

677
Don't starve
If you save up all your calories for alcohol by not eating before going out, you're more likely to grab high-calorie snacks after having a few

drinks—alcohol causes blood-sugar levels to drop, which tells your brain you're hungry.

678
Eat before you go

Before you get to a party, have a banana and a glass of skim milk or a chicken sandwich on whole wheat bread. Your judgment and willpower will then be greater when faced with chips or champagne.

679
Drink with a meal

The most beneficial way to drink is with a sit-down meal, placing the bottle in the middle of the table so you can see how much you've drunk.

680
Red salsa

Offer this to guests with raw vegetables for dipping.

2 small red onions, finely chopped
2 green chiles, finely chopped
8 ripe tomatoes, chopped
bunch of fresh cilantro leaves
2 limes
sea salt and black pepper, to season

Combine the onions, chiles, and tomatoes in a bowl. Finely chop the cilantro and stir in. Squeeze the limes and stir in the juice. Season.

681
Tasty crudité dip

Take 9oz (250g) of smoked mackerel and 9oz (250g) of low-fat cream cheese. Process in a blender with 3 tbsp fresh parsley and a squeeze of lemon juice.

682
Eat Japanese

The traditional Japanese diet gains its health benefits from being largely based on rice and grains, fish, seafood, and sea vegetables—and by cutting out fatty animal and dairy products. Buy a teach-yourself recipe book.

683
Avoid pillow packs

Pre-packaged salad leaves in modified-atmosphere packaging

Learn to cook Japanese food and enjoy a healthy low-fat diet.

may have lower levels of antioxidant nutrients including vitamin C. For maximum nutrients choose fresh lettuces, and wash them yourself.

684
Serve small and big

Provide masses of undressed salads at a buffet accompanied by small portions of higher-fat foods, such as smoked salmon, cheese, and meats.

685
Make your own dressings

To mix your own, combine 1 part balsamic vinegar to 6 parts extra-virgin olive oil, a squeeze of lemon juice, pinch of herbs de Provence, twist of black pepper, and ½–1 tsp each of mustard and honey.

686
Indulge

Choose foods that feel naughty, but are relatively low in calories and packed with protein, vitamins, and minerals, such as lobster, crab, shrimp, and mussels.

687
Take it home

When eating out, ask for a doggie bag rather than trying to finish every bit of food on the table, and take home untouched dishes.

688
Juicy fruits

Pile some of the following into a pretty dish—the jewel-like colors

Indulgent food isn't always unhealthy: lobster is rich in vitamins, minerals, and protein.

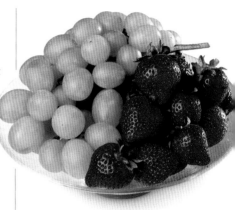

Pile small fresh fruits into a pretty dish to create an appetizing starter.

look pretty and appetizing:
- Red and green grapes
- Red-, white-, and blackcurrants
- Different colored melon slices
- Raspberries and strawberries
- Blueberries

689
Perfect present

If you really enjoy a local wine, ask for part of the vineyard as a birthday gift. You may be allocated 12 or so trees and the chance to help out at grape-picking time as well as a case of that year's vintage.

690
Healthy party gifts

Try these alternatives to a box of chocolates or bottle of champagne:
- Pots of herbs
- Vouchers for tennis lessons
- An apple or cherry tree
- First pressing of a fine olive oil

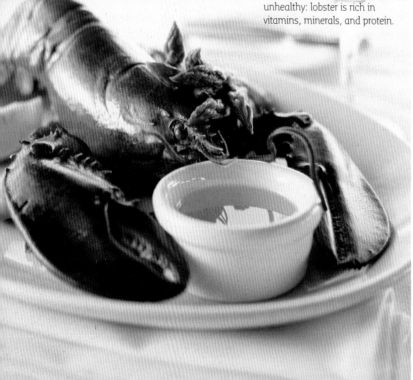

Dancing into shape

Dance is such a valuable way of keeping in shape because once you're in the groove, you forget you're doing it. And you don't have to go to the gym to benefit. Whether you dance in the kitchen as you cook, with your toddler at a play session, or in a club on a Saturday night, dancing keeps many body systems in shape, from circulation and respiration to the skeletal-muscular and nervous systems.

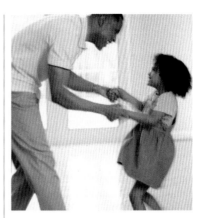

Dance with your child at play sessions and burn calories while you are at it.

691
Find a style to suit you
There's a form of dance for every type of body and level of fitness and commitment, from technically precise ballet to freeform Five Rhythms. Find your perfect match by trying sampler classes, watching DVDs or live shows, and seeking out music you adore.

692
Take your partner
Ballroom dancing is perfect if you haven't exercised for some time or you like learning a skill. By building one-to-one relationships, it acts as an antidote to the social isolation that keeps many, especially older, people in sedentary lifestyles.

693
Learn a move from an elder
Plunder unlikely sources for dance moves. How did your grandfather dance as a young man? Ask him to show you a move. Can you volunteer at a retirement home exercise session or dance class for older people? What tricks can they teach you?

694
Wind up a phonograph
Buy or borrow an old-fashioned wind-up phonograph and dig around in your granny's attic or online for 78rpm records. Head off to a quiet beach or park with some friends, and make up dances to the tunes (or take granny with you and have her show you how to foxtrot!).

695
Which shoes to choose?
For beginners and professionals alike, wearing the right shoes is essential to good technique and safety. Shape, heel size, and circumference vary according to style of dance, so take advice from a teacher. Rounded toes allow the feet to spread, for better balance and posture. Good-quality leather gets less sweaty than synthetics and molds to the foot. For different-sized feet, look for made-to-measure shoes.

696
Safe landing
Before jumping, practice landing safely: land on the balls of your feet, bending your knees, then transfer your weight to your heels. Aim for silence. Bad landings are not just noisy, they jar the spine.

697
Warming up
To prevent injury and connect your mind with your body, start to dance by slowly writing your name in space using different parts of your body: try your nose, hips, and big toes. This is also good for areas recovering from injury.

698
Spatial awareness visualization

This is a good warm-up for all dancers. Spot four points in space (don't confine yourself to the floor). Make up and memorize a flowing sequence of movements during which you "touch" each spot with a different part of your body.

699
Music warm-up

Put on some music you love and dance for 5 minutes to increase your body temperature. Once you feel slightly breathless, warm up your joints by focusing your movements on one area of the body in turn: dance from your hips, knees, ankles, and toes, then your shoulders, wrists, and fingers.

700
Group dancing

If you like to exercise with friends, consider street-dance classes or line dancing. Both include group routines that give the heart and lungs a good workout as well as developing coordination and poise.

701
Your body in space

When warming up, spend time in all planes: remember that you can move up and down, side to side, and backward as well as forward. Give in to gravity, too, by exploring prone and supine positions on the floor.

Join a dance group with your friends; then you can have fun with them while you work out.

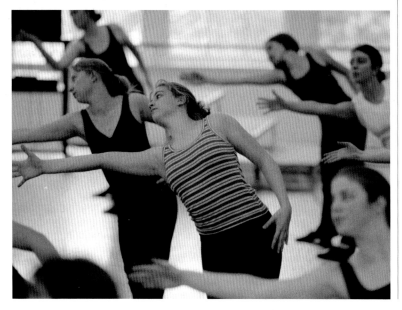

702
Align your joints

Before you begin any form of dance, stand and check your alignment, positioning your head over your shoulders, your shoulders over your hips, your hips over your knees, and knees over your heels. Relax your shoulders and open your chest as if opening a book (your spine being the book's spine). Well-aligned bones lead to easy movement and reduce the risk of injury, especially on the joints, while an open chest permits deeper breathing, which oxygenates your tissues so that they can work at maximum efficiency.

703
Get a massage

In a 1999 study, dance students who had twice-weekly massages for one month found they had an increased range of motion, improved balance and posture, and decreased levels of the stress hormone cortisol.

704
Hydration matters

If you dance vigorously enough to sweat, ensure you get enough essential fatty acids in your diet: they equip your body to hold on to water. Find them in linseed (flaxseed), rapeseed (canola), and walnut oils. Apply evening primrose and wheatgerm oils during massage.

705

Pilates warm-up

Many dancers use Pilates exercises to warm up and speed rehabilitation after injury. The exercises lengthen and strengthen muscles in a balanced way, and focus on mobilizing joints as well as stabilizing the core muscles that hold you upright.

706

Attitude and passion

Take heart if you are older: the best flamenco dancers tend to be older women whose expertise comes not only through practice, but life experience. Flamenco offers the whole body a powerful workout, while learning the rhythms also keeps the brain in good shape.

707

End of evening wind-down

At the end of an evening session, lie on your back with legs and arms spread, palms up. Tense your feet and calves and hold your breath. Exhale and let go, feeling your feet and legs relax. Repeat up your body from thighs to shoulders. Finally, scrunch up your face and neck. Let it go. Rest for 5 to 10 minutes, feeling how good relaxation is after tension.

Flamenco asks you to invest passion and ditch your reserve: where else are you encouraged to stamp your feet in public?

Sweat-free reshaping

If boot camps, privation, and endurance sports aren't your thing, spend your leisure time on activities that make a difference to the way you look and feel without the pain, from a good haircut to a slimming body wrap. But do keep up the healthy eating and don't forget to get some physical exercise most days: it has been said that taking no exercise is equivalent to smoking a pack of cigarettes each day.

708

Perfect your posture

When you stand tall, you look leaner. Stand with feet hip-width apart and distribute your body weight evenly over both feet. Sway from side to side and back to front to check. Lengthen up from this grounded standing position, pulling up through your ankles, knees, and thighs and weighting the base of your spine as if you have a kangaroo tail. Lift your shoulders to your ears, then drop them without losing length in your sides. Finally, lengthen the back of your neck: imagine the crown of your head being pulled up by a balloon.

709

Reshape your hair

Try a salon "reshaping" or deep-conditioning treatment to bring body, shine, and swing to lifeless or hard-to-manage hair.

710

Body reshaping

Relax while pads or a belt are strapped around areas of flab—tummy, thighs, hips, tops of arms. When switched on, electrical impulses stimulate muscle fibers for increased firmness. A 20-minute session is said to be worth 350 sit-ups.

711

Vibrate it away

Buy a power plate vibration platform and keep it by the phone; stand on it while taking calls and boost muscle tone.

712

Go as a couple

Look for spas that offer a couple experience, where you can share twin baths, side-by-side massage

Find a spa that offers a couple experience, and work on your relationship as well as your body.

(often with four therapists), romantic candlelit facials, and champagne pedicures before retiring to a rose-petal-strewn bed. This beats chocolates for a Valentine treat.

713
Contour wraps

Lie back and relax as a beauty therapist smothers you in clay, plant, or marine products, and then wraps you in bandages or plastic and maybe heats your skin, too. Many salon or spa body-mask treatments claim inch-loss results.

714
Hip and thigh treatments

Salon treatments for the hips and thighs can leave them feeling smoother and possibly more taut. Over about an hour, expect to be dry-brushed, exfoliated, massaged, wrapped in detoxifying products, cleansed, and moisturized.

715
Visit a thermal spa

Taking to the water has been valued as a way of reshaping body, mind, and soul since pre-Roman times. Visit an ancient spa town to luxuriate in naturally heated waters and drink mineral water that is considered healing and rejuvenating, or visit a modern thermal bath park.

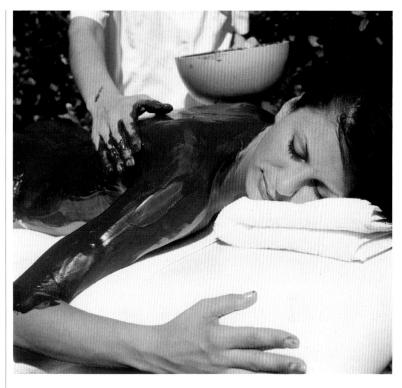

Lie back and lose inches: many body-mask treatments claim size-reduction benefits.

716
Soak in vitality

Spa vitality pools resemble huge Jacuzzis; boost your circulation with a swim, then move to one of the "massage stations," including bubble airbeds or shooting water geysers, where strategic jets pummel your flab underwater.

717
Room with a view

If your gym looks out over the sea or has an eagle-eye view of the city, you may feel more motivated during exercise sessions. To find one that encourages this approach, look for statues of the Buddha, soft lighting, and meditation or chill-out rooms.

718
Leave time to sleep

Getting a healthy amount of sleep is one of the keys to losing weight and keeping it off. So, alongside sleep-health workshops or sleep yoga, high-end spas are introducing luxury sleeping rooms or snooze zones, featuring CDs of white noise and MP3 players pre-loaded with sleep programming. When booking a treatment or class, build in time for a snooze afterward.

719

Enjoy a mud massage

Take a partner for a Moroccan-inspired *rhassoul* treatment. In a eucalyptus-scented steamy room, you massage each other with mineral-rich mud, then relax on heated thrones as the steam opens your pores. The session finishes with a shower from the roof.

720

Hot stone massage

After a deep-tissue massage, a LaStone therapist applies heated and frozen stones to tune up the major chakras—subtle energy points described in the yogic tradition sited at seven points along the spine. This is thought to undo blockages in the invisible energy channels that criss-cross the body, bringing about a greater sense of well-being in mind, emotions, and body.

721

Zero balancing

In this very gentle form of touch therapy, you lie on a massage table as a therapist exerts pressure with her fingers around your bones and joints to release deep-held tension and rebalance the flow of your subtle energy, or life-force. This is thought to help your body "reorganize" itself, which results in improved posture, a feeling of lightness, strength, and refreshment, and easier movement.

722

Let someone take over

Choose a weight-loss spa break not only to lose a pound or two, but also to be handed life-changing exercise, dietary, and lifestyle solutions on a plate.

723

Home bodywrap

This home detox treatment can be effective for problem areas, such as the thighs, tummy, and tops of the arms. Use it in a very warm room. Avoid during pregnancy or if you have vascular problems.

- 1 very ripe papaya
- 5 tbsp fine oatmeal
- 1 tbsp honey
- 1 tbsp aloe vera gel
- 1 cup green tea, for mixing
- 4 drops each essential oils of lavender and juniper

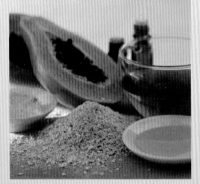

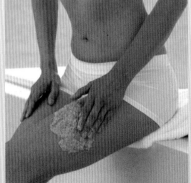

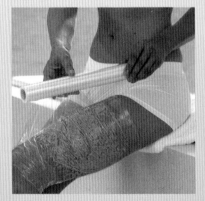

1 In a blender, mix the papaya flesh with the oatmeal. Mix in the honey, aloe vera gel, and enough green tea to make a fine paste. Stir in the oils.

2 Exfoliate your "problem" area with a body brush, always stroking toward the heart, then smear the clay liberally over the area.

3 Wrap in plastic wrap (not over-tight), then warmed towels, and relax for 30 minutes. Unwrap, rinse off the clay, and moisturize.

Get active outdoors

Escape into the great outdoors—the green gym—and exercise becomes more holistic, inspiring your spirit and calming your mind while toning your muscles. In one study, 72 percent of green gym participants were still active after six months—you can't say that for many gym memberships.

724

Join a green gym

Although there are set warm-up and cool-down routines in a "green gym," there are no gym-like exercises. You get fit by helping to conserve the landscape (usually in a country park or wildlife sanctuary)—cutting back undergrowth, making paths, and building dry-stone walls, hedging or planting trees, with all the walking, carrying, and digging such tasks involve. The activities change with the seasons and as you work, you learn about biodiversity and habitat, and the history of the landscape or species you're helping to conserve. The biggest buzz is not the noticeable effects on body and mind or the close friendships forged, but the tangible results on the landscape.

725

Country garden exercise

The grounds of many country houses or gardens feature trails suited to different levels of fitness and ability, from wheelchair tracks and one-mile beginner walks to high-energy hill climbs. Some doctors may be able to enroll you on a leisure-walking program that offers free entry and a guide.

Walk with the seasons and savor the differences as the months roll by.

726

Seasonal fun

Plan walks that change with the seasons—find circular trails that take in spring blossom, bluebell woods, displays of autumn foliage, and early morning winter frosting.

727

Walk a barefoot trail

Outdoor barefoot walking trails are popular in Germany and China, and 2005 research showed that walking over their various-textured surfaces for 30 minutes three times a week for four months improved balance and blood pressure. Make a barefoot trail in your garden by laying down garden canes, gravel and pebbles, crunchy leaves and bark chippings, soft sand, cold water, and even mud. Take off your shoes and walk over each surface very slowly.

728
Country walk

On the weekend, appreciate the countryside in which your food grows by planning out a walk that passes a farm shop or farm-gate stall. As you walk, notice how the methods of cultivation and choice of

Attend open days teaching grow your own techniques for individual crops such as chiles.

crop or livestock have molded the look of the countryside, and point this out to children to help them make the connection between what they eat and where it grows.

729
Watch the birdie

In the spring, take a walk in local woodlands or reed-beds as the sun rises to see how many birdsongs you can recognize. Dawn-chorus walks organized by experts help novices learn to identify calls, and improve fitness while they are at it.

730
No time to walk?

Walk at night, when work and housework are over and children are in bed. Is there a full-moon or women's nightwalking group in your area? Try to walk in silence, at least one way, to better experience night's different sounds and textures. There is safety in numbers, so take a friend.

731
Learn country crafts

Country crafts sessions using native materials get you out into the countryside gathering materials before teaching the intellectual skills and body know-how to work them into beautiful objects. Look for courses in basket-weaving, building

willow structures, rope-making, carving greenwood furniture, or hedgerow winemaking.

732
"Grow your own" day

Open days at organic farms and agricultural colleges offer outdoor talks, demonstrations, and hands-on guides to cultivating vegetables. Sometimes there's a focus on one crop, such as chiles or onions, with resident experts, and at other venues, you get to cook and eat the produce.

733
Try a conservation vacation

Visit some of the finest landscapes in the world and help to conserve them as you tone up, whether working on sites of classical heritage in Albania, doing coastal work to benefit birds in Bulgaria, or conserving the habitat of endangered primates in Cameroon. Accommodation is often simple and you have to help out with cooking, but that only adds to the sense of adventure. To find opportunities, look at The National Wildlife Federation's website at www.nwf.org.

734
Active learning

A 2004 review of research found that getting away from a book and computer-based setting enhances learning. Being active in a

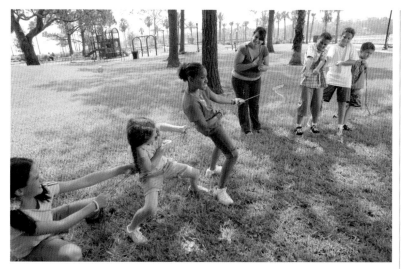

If you live in the city, find out about activities taking place in local parks and join in.

memorable place has an especially positive impact on long-term fact-retention: the more senses you use as you learn, the more of the brain that is employed in retaining memory. If you are studying, get into the great outdoors to shape up your cognitive skills.

735
Wilderness therapy
Encourage kids to take part in outdoor activity camps and trips to wild places. A 2006 review of research concluded that wilderness experiences are very important for a child's physical, emotional, cognitive and mental, and social development. Being in extreme places seems to forge long-lasting behavioral changes by forcing young people to think responsibly, look after themselves, and protect others.

736
Grown-ups' summer camp
Don't let kids have all the fun — surprise them by booking yourself into an activity camp this summer. Ease in gently with a yoga or t'ai chi camp, which offers teachers from diverse schools of practice and early-morning and late-night sessions. A hiking camp with dawn-to-dusk guided walks may suit more seasoned exercisers, although even these include gentle rambles and nature-watching sessions suitable for novices.

737
Take a city stroll
If you don't live near the countryside, you can still exercise in a green way. Buy a guidebook or download a city walk that takes in handsome buildings, industrial heritage sites, rivers, parks, and cathedrals. If there's a tower, climb the steps to the top for a panoramic view.

738
Celebrate seasonal fare
In town, seek out seasonal festivals celebrating the harvest. On apple days, sample local varieties and take part in apple-bobbing games; at a tomato festival, sign up for a fruit-throwing contest; at eggplant or onion time, enjoy speciality dishes and dancing till dawn.

739
City park fitness
If you like being pushed to achieve your best, look for army vets teaching fitness sessions in city parks. In addition to push-ups, instructors include team-building games such as tug of war, and participants are graded by ability, with fitness-focused, weight-loss, and team-building options.

740
Scavenger hunt
Join a team to run around town or countryside for a day or weekend searching for items on a list and photographing them, or performing extreme (often embarrassing) tasks—and being taped in the act. The first to finish or the team with the most objects wins.

Self-powered sports

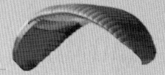

The more you power activities with your body, the more muscle-mass you build; the more muscle you have, the more calories your body burns, even at rest. Sports powered by you—or by the tide, wind, or sun—are also perhaps the greenest sports of all, helping to keep the planet in shape, too.

741

Being energetic builds muscle

For best muscle-building benefit, choose activities that strength-train the large muscles that power most of your movement—in your thighs, chest, and abdominals—such as rowing, cycling, and cross-country skiing. Aim for 30 minutes of this type of resistance training weekly.

742

Try Zen archery

Muscle-building sports are more effective if you maintain focused awareness as you train. To learn this skill, try a session of Zen archery, *kyudo*, in which shooting an arrow is regarded as a moving meditation.

743

Take a short break

Keep your carbon footprint small by seeking out sports powered by you that you can enjoy close to home. Look for a multi-activity adventure weekend, where you dabble in a number of sports, from climbing to paragliding and blo-karting.

744

Try a Brazilian martial art

If your lack of upper-body strength bothers you, learn a skill that pushes you to have more confidence in your arms, wrists, and shoulders. Capoeira is one of the best: it requires stamina, flexibility, and leg power, but upper-body strength is key to the cartwheel and handstand movements. For many women, the emphasis on push-ups is empowering because practice brings results. And having the confidence to

show your skills in the *roda*, or ring, empowers you to succeed in cooperative sports, such as climbing.

745

Indoor climbing

City climbing walls have opened up the sport of climbing. Don't worry if

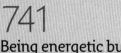

you lack upper-body muscle—climbing is more coordination, balance, and technique than brute strength, and you learn to rely on legs and feet over arms and fingers.

746
Join a climbing club

The best way to start climbing outdoors is to join a local climbing club. You may be expected to have your own gear as well as a good grasp of basic skills, but you will benefit from organized trips to crags as well as meeting potential climbing partners.

747
Climbers' warm-up

To stretch key parts of the body that need to stay flexible when you climb, get onto all fours, then straighten your arms and push your buttocks back and toward the sky (Downward Dog—see No. 186). Raise one leg and bend at the knee to swing the whole leg and hip back. If you can, twist over and place your foot on the ground, then pick up the same-side hand and stretch it back, thrusting your pelvis to the sky. Turn back to Downward Dog and repeat with the other leg.

748
Bouldering

This is a less daunting option than mountain climbing: you climb close to the ground on low-lying rocks. Bouldering allows you to work on your form, practice independently, and learn sequences and solutions.

749
Conquering fear

A surprising number of climbers have a fear of heights or of falling. If this is holding you back, try a consultation with an NLP

Try sports such as paragliding that require little more than nature to power you along.

(Neuro-Linguistic Programming) practitioner. Learn meditation, too, to keep you focused on the moment.

750
Caving and potholing
If you like climbing but don't have a head for heights, explore caving. Join a caving club and let experts guide you through the basics.

751
Ski-prep exercise
Skiing can be an exhilarating form of exercise. Be sure to prepare your muscles before you take to the slopes. Place your lower back against a wall with feet a foot forward. Press your lower back into the wall and slide down until you feel a stretch in your thigh muscles (keep knees over ankles). For extra work, pin your shoulder blades to the wall and stretch your arms overhead.

752
Ski thinking
Practice focusing your brain on your legs as you work through ski-preparation exercises—this is where it needs to stay while you are skiing.

753
Take a break
If you push yourself in sports or competitions, make sure you take weekly recovery days to rest your joints and preserve enough energy to give your best on training days.

754
Monitor your training
Wearing a heart-rate monitor allows you to push yourself to your limits of aerobic endurance and helps you maintain peak effort when other factors, such as wind-speed, change.

755
Serious sports stretch
This yoga sequence suits extreme sports fanatics who are already toned and helps to develop the attitude you need to accomplish mean feats.

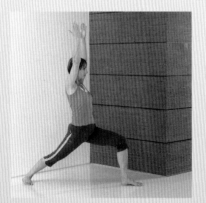
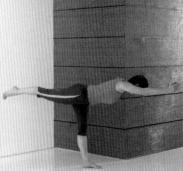

1 Stand with your feet wide apart and stretch your arms overhead. Twist your feet, hips, and chest left and bend your left leg, trying to make a right angle with your front knee.

2 Stretch forward over your left thigh, raise your back foot, and straighten your front leg to make a "T" shape. Come back down. Repeat Steps 1 and 2 to the other side.

3 Place your hands on the floor, shoulder-width apart, near a support. Walk your feet in, then kick your legs up into a supported handstand. Repeat 3 times.

756
Heart-rate calculations
To establish your maximum heart rate, subtract your age from 226 for women and 220 for men. This indicates the maximum number of beats per minute during training if you are mostly sedentary. Once you get more active, subtract half your age from 205.

757
How are you progressing?
Gauge how well your heart is shaping up over a few months by monitoring your resting heart rate with a monitor, perhaps on waking. As your heart muscle tones up, it will be able to beat more powerfully, requiring fewer beats per minute to pump blood around your body.

758
Power eating
If you strength train for 45 minutes or more three days a week, check that you are eating protein daily, and have a protein-rich snack an hour or so before training.

759
An apple a day
Take an apple to munch as a break from extreme activities to boost your lung function (the more efficiently your lungs work, the more oxygen is available for your cells and the better your ability to expel airborne toxins).

760
Sun loving
It's tricky to get out of the sun when hanging off a rock face or competing in a half-marathon. Protect your skin by wearing an organic sunblock and cover up with thick cotton layers, sunglasses, and a wide-brimmed hat if possible.

761
Eat colorfully
Fruit and vegetables high in plant nutrients known as carotenoids offer skin some protection from UV light, as do the polyphenols in green tea and sulphoraphane in broccoli.

762
Carotenoid fruit salad
For a UV-protecting breakfast, slice and mix together a combination of the following fruits: cantaloupe, mango, nectarines, papaya, and fresh or dried (soaked) apricots.

763
Care for your joints
If you're unused to physical activity, a sudden surge of intensity increases the likelihood of an injury in the body's largest joints, the knees and hips. To keep them in good working order, especially as you age, warm up well before starting extreme activity, and cool down well afterward.

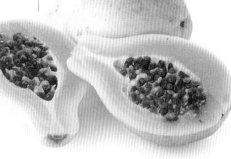

Papaya contains carotenoids which help protect skin against UV damage.

764
Homeopathic remedies
The following may help to ease back pain brought on by extreme activity:
• Hypericum 30: for injuries to the spine caused by jarring movements.
• Bryonia 30: for a seized-up back, when the slightest movement is intensely painful.
• Aesculus 30: for injuries to the sacral area, or sacroiliac joints.

765
Mint tonic foot soak
Place 2 tbsp of dried mint in a mug and pour just-boiled water overtop. Allow to steep for 20 minutes before straining into a footbath.

Coastal fun

You don't have to be an extreme sports enthusiast to gain body benefits from spending time at the coast. Research into the effects of thalassotherapy, or seawater treatments, show that simply staying in a marine environment enhances peace of mind, sleep quality, and the ability to deal with stressful situations; it also increases energy levels and self-confidence. All are essentials in your shaping-up kit.

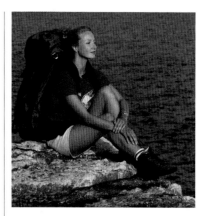

Take a break and reduce stress simply by sitting and staring out to sea.

766
Breathe in ocean air
A study of people with health problems at Dead Sea resorts in Israel found that their breathing improved thanks to the high levels of salt and minerals in the atmosphere, and the low altitude (which produces air 10 percent richer in oxygen than at regular sea-level). Look for low-lying seaside resorts and practice breathing exercises on the beach to shape up your lungs.

Tone the muscles in your lower limbs and improve balance by walking on soft sand.

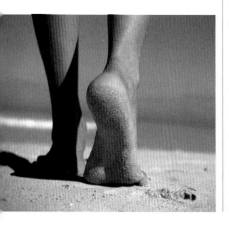

767
Sit and stare
One study found that the quickest way to cut stress for most people was to look at the ocean. To keep your mind and emotions in shape, how often could you visit the coast?

768
Walk the coastline
Many coasts feature marked cliff-top walks. For the more adventurous, complete a coast-to-coast walk or circumnavigate a peninsula in sections over various weekends through the year.

769
Take a meditation walk
Book a coastal meditation walk with a yoga teacher: being high above the landscape and within sight and sound of the ever-crashing waves can be a source of support at times of mental stress or emotional burnout.

770
Coasteering
This is the art of traversing a coastal area or rocky shore by feet, hands, and water. It's a great way of getting fit, since you walk, swim, scramble, climb, and abseil or cliff-jump to explore inaccessible coves and caves. Go with a guide—you can book half- or full-day packages (complete with wetsuit and safety helmet) and ecotours that feature dolphin and seal watching.

771
Sand walking
Walking on soft sand challenges the muscles in your lower limbs and your balance, requiring greater effort to keep you upright and moving forward. This gives a better cardio workout than walking on dry land and increases toning (and calorie burning).

772
Castles in the sand

Organize a sandcastle competition for children or adults. Set a theme (mermaids, fantasy palaces, creatures from the deep), a time-frame, and award prizes for the most innovative. Encourage younger children to help by beachcombing for decorative materials, from feathers for flags to seaweed for mermaid's hair.

773
Sea swimming

When you swim in the ocean (without wearing a wet suit), you expose your skin to the antiseptic properties of seawater, used to treat dermatitis, psoriasis, and skin allergies because it promotes healing, relieves itching and inflammation, and boosts immunity.

774
Go bare

Dare to try a nudist beach—often the most beautiful because they are hidden from view. It's liberating to be freed from the tyranny of ill-fitting bikinis—size and shape aren't an issue at nudist resorts.

775
Pick mussels

Wild mussels aren't as big as those in fish markets, but the flavor is memorable. Pick at low tide, choosing mussels from rocks covered by the tide twice a day and out of the range of sewage outlets. Avoid open mussels that don't close when tapped. Leave in a bucket of cold seawater in a cool place for a couple of hours to dislodge sand and grit, then pull off the "beard" and cook immediately.

776
Mussels with shallots and cream

Pick a supermarket-sized bag of mussels, clean (see No. 775), and place in a pot with a lid. Add 2–3 finely chopped shallots and a glass of white wine, bring to a boil, and simmer for 3 minutes, covered, until the mussels open (discard those that don't). Stir in a couple of tablespoons of cream (and a handful of chopped parsley if you have it) and eat with fresh bread.

777
Clam bake

Clams are rich in potassium, a mineral most of us are deficient in. Hold a clam bake on the beach. You can also wrap potatoes or sweet potatoes in foil to bake in the embers

Build sandcastles to stimulate creativity and imagination as well as increasing activity on the beach.

of the fire, serving them with a yogurt dip: potatoes and yogurt are also good sources of potassium.

778
Sea-beet and chickpeas

This salad of wild sea greens is delicious served with new potatoes and easy to make in one pan over a beach fire or camping stove. Identify the sea beet using a forager's guide.

1 onion, finely chopped
2 pieces Canadian bacon, cut into slices
1 tsp garam masala
2 handfuls sea beet, washed and chopped
1 x 240g can chickpeas (pre-cooked and drained)
1 x 240g can plum tomatoes, chopped
sea salt and black pepper, to taste

Cook the onion in a large pan until soft and translucent, then add the bacon and cook through. Stir in the garam masala and cook until fragrant, then add the sea beet and cook until wilted. Pour in the chickpeas and tomatoes, and let bubble until warmed through. Season to taste and serve immediately. Serves 2.

779
Catch your dinner

Book a day on a line-fishing boat and expend calories catching your dinner. Some boats offer "hook and cook" days, where you learn basic cooking techniques aboard ship.

780
Baywatch safety

If you live near the coast, enroll older children in a sea-safety course. Led by qualified lifeguards and adventure instructors, they will learn about the dangers of the ocean and basic surf rescue as well as exploring the marine life in rock pools.

781
Rock pool adventuring

For rock-pooling with a twist, stay up late and go out with a full moon. Wear a head flashlight to keep your hands free, and read a tide timetable so you know when to anticipate the return of the sea.

782
Learn to crew

By taking a competent crew course, in five days you can learn to crew a cruising yacht, understanding how to man the helm, tie knots, forecast wind and weather, and handle sails.

Eating sea fish you have caught yourself makes a nutritious, eco-friendly, and satisfying dinner.

Cool camping tips

A camping trip is a calorie-loss trip. The sun wakes you early when you sleep under canvas, forcing you to get up and be active from early in the morning, and even the smallest of daily tasks—going to the bathroom, washing up—require a few hundred steps across a field. Campers also spend many happy hours squatting and sitting on the floor, which tones the thighs, buttocks, and lower back.

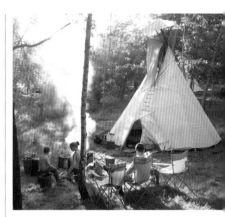

Enjoy the benefits of camping without the stress by hiring a ready-assembled tent.

783
One-pot cooking
The essence of easy eating on camp is one-pot meals. Before you go, scour your cookbooks and the Internet for two or three robust dishes for which exact ingredients don't matter—casseroles, curries, and chunky soups are all good choices. Take the ingredients with you or prepare part of the dish in advance to spare cooking gas and kindling on site.

784
Camp kitchen essentials
Don't forget the following to enliven throw-together camp meals:
• Fresh chiles and bottles of hot chile sauce
• Fresh lemons
• Garlic
• Dried herbes de Provence
• Olive oil and balsamic vinegar
• Soy sauce
• Wine, sherry, or cider for cooking

785
Make your own cheese
Impress the campsite by making your own low-fat cheese overnight. Heat a few pints of milk (unpasteurized if you can buy it) to boiling point, then add the juice of a lemon and a pinch of salt. Continue to heat, stirring, and watch the milk separate into curds (lumps) and whey (liquid). Let the milk cool, then pour into a piece of muslin (cheesecloth) and tie securely. Swing the muslin around your head

Take garlic with you on camping trips as it is a key camp kitchen ingredient.

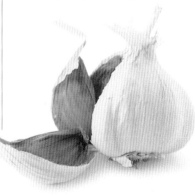

until all the liquid has been forced out, then hang from a branch overnight. Ease out of the muslin next morning and spread on toast.

786
Dandelion salad
During spring camping, pick the first few dandelion leaves as they start to shoot and use them as a tasty addition to a green salad. The flavor combines well with just-cooked bacon, but be sure to scatter the bacon over the salad just before serving and dressing to prevent wilting.

787
Luxury camping
You don't even have to be able to pitch a tent to go camping. Look for a site where you can hire a ready-assembled tent—perhaps a tepee or Mongolian yurt, with wood-burning stove and feather beds.

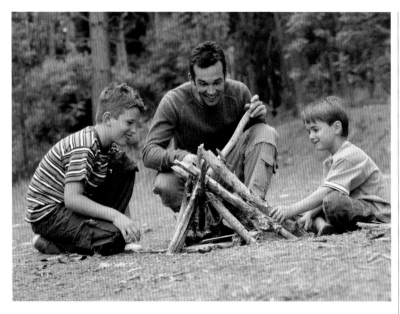

Get back to nature and learn basic survival skills with your children at a family eco camp.

792
Rainy-day games
When you're stuck in a tent with restless campers, try these games:
- Slug races (circle the tent in a sleeping bag)
- Cat's cradle (string finger games)
- Singing
- Make an outfit from newspaper
- Origami
- Prepare an activity for another tent, then swap tents

793
Yoga for comfy sitting
In your tent, sit back to back with a partner. If necessary, sit the shorter partner on a cushion. Pull your feet toward your groin and let your knees relax to the sides. Breathe deeply, feeling the breath running up and down your partner's spine.

788
Family eco camps
To boost your outdoor confidence, study survival skills with the experts at an eco camp. You'll learn how to start a fire and keep it going, alternative ways to make a shelter, and ways to find and cook food.

789
Camp fitness game
Shuffle a pack of cards and allocate exercises to each suit: diamonds might be sit-ups, hearts jumping jacks, spades push-ups, and clubs squats. Take turns picking a card and complete the number of exercises shown. Aces count as 21! When you pick a king, queen, or jack, take a 60-second recovery walk.

790
Play Frisbee
Running, throwing, and leaping to catch a Frisbee builds cardiovascular fitness and endurance.

791
Practice catching
Try a Frisbee "crocodile" catch—extend both arms in front of you and try to catch the disc between your palms by snapping them shut, like the jaws of a croc.

Be prepared for all climates by taking wet-weather activities like origami with you.

794
Take a belt
For easy sitting at camp, take a yoga belt. Sit cross-legged and secure the

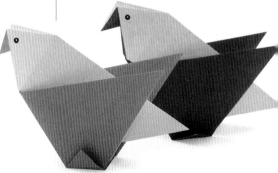

strap around your knees and lower back, pulling it tight enough to act as a reassuring brace.

795
Remedies for bites and stings

Life in the open air means sharing your space with other creatures; here are homeopathic remedies to deal with the consequences:

• Apis 30: made from the sting of the honey bee, which is exactly what it antidotes.

• Ledum 30: reduces the maddening itch of insect bites.

• Urtica Urens 30: made from nettles, the stings of which it treats, as well as other itchy rashes caused by plants or allergies.

796
Sunburn treatment

Take a homeopathic first aid kit on camping trips. It should contain Belladonna 30, which works wonders for sunburn and the throbbing headache associated with sunstroke. If the sunburn is threatening to blister, take Cantharis 30 to promote rapid healing.

797
Sunburn flower remedy

The flowers of the desert plant Mulla Mulla are a head of red spiky petals covered in white hairs, giving the appearance of flames and smoke. The Australian Bush Flower Essence made from this plant treats burns, including sunburn, as well as emotional trauma caused by injury from fire or the sun.

798
Sleeping-bag stargazing

When it gets dark, put down a ground sheet and place your sleeping bags in a row; lie back and look at the night sky. If you have a star chart or someone who knows the names of constellations, point them out. If not, make up stories about the pictures you can see when you join the dots.

799
Camp treasure hunt

Send children off into the undergrowth to hunt for leaves from six different trees and find stones from three types of rock. On their return, provide them with tree and mineral identification guides so they can put names to them. Children who feel at home outdoors are more likely to become active adults.

Involve your community

It's easiest to stay in shape if those around you are doing the same. Some projects show just how life-changing shaping up in your community can be: for example, community garden projects bring together the benefits of physical activity and a healthy diet, the therapeutic effects of gardening, and greater social interaction to all who join them.

800
Community gardens

Transforming weed-infested dumps into places to grow food or flowers is good for the mental health of a whole community, suggest programs that do just that. They seem to act as a focal point for informal social interaction, which makes people feel safer outdoors. This increased sense of well-being also encourages residents to step outside to exercise. Is there a space you could reclaim?

801
School grounds

Why not join a committee to improve your local school grounds? There is good evidence that getting involved in school-grounds projects develops community cohesion and also encourages children to spend more time being active outdoors. Indeed, it may be the only space they have for safe outdoor play. You could raise funds toward climbing and play equipment, dig up overgrown borders to create mini plots for each class, or plan a sensory garden.

802
Clean-up week

Is there a beach clean-up or street-cleaning week where you live? Can you start one? Everyone benefits when you make your community a better place to live, and volunteers get fitter in the process.

803
Get everyone involved

If you're planning a project to transform a piece of wasteland or to canvass for more sporting facilities, try an approach that worked well in Scotland: set up a sticky board or "graffiti wall" in a prominent place such as a shopping mall, and ask passers-by to stick notes or drawings to it expressing their opinions. For food projects, give out paper plates and have people draw what they'd like to be able to buy and where.

804
Walking the dog

If you don't want the hassle of taking care of a dog, but could use an excuse to walk every day, start a dog-walking service in your area, either voluntary or paid.

805
Train as a leader

Does your health authority run a program that trains volunteers to lead walks around your locality, including walks prescribed by doctors in "walking for health" programs? You'll get fit while learning leadership skills and ways to keep fellow walkers motivated.

806
Gardening as therapy

By stimulating all the senses, horticultural therapy helps keep memory skills in shape and boosts a sense of connection to a place or community. It also counters loneliness, isolation, and depression. Ask your doctor about projects.

807
Blog your veg

To keep up your motivation for gardening, set up your own

Start up a local dog-walking service to get you walking every day.

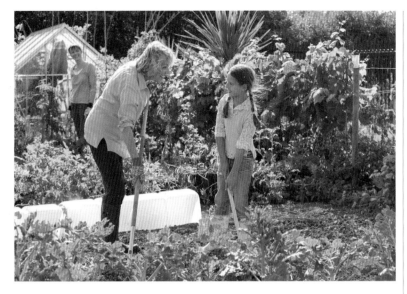

Counter loneliness and boost memory by participating in a community garden project.

gardening blog to join an online community of gardeners. Read http://americanheir loomgardener. blogspot.com for inspiration: follow the links to top gardening blogs.

808
Supermarket tours
Is there a free supermarket tour in your town given by a health group? They help community groups to understand how food is labeled and how to "read" the supermarket layout to find healthier foods.

809
Join a food co-op
A food co-op buys fresh, whole (often local) food in bulk and sells it direct, maybe at wholesale price, to local people. People who join co-ops tend to eat more fresh produce and more variety, including seasonal foods that are too delicate, ripe, or misshapen for supermarkets. Your local authority or organic growers' association might run a course to help you set up a group. Indirect benefits include getting out and about, making new friends (including isolated farmers), and learning about how food is grown and seasonal availability.

810
Organize a potluck meal
At the beginning and end of a community project, organize a community meal, asking everyone who is involved to each bring one home-cooked dish. Invite children to join in the preparation of the meal to evangelize the fun of cooking and sharing food in groups. Play board games after clearing away the plates.

811
Wield a wooden spoon
Love cooking? Fed up that younger people don't recognize regional dishes, cooking techniques, or raw ingredients? Speak to your local authority about Get Cooking programs that can fund you to run cooking classes.

812
Write a cookbook
Compile a recipe book with your local school or worship group. Include recipes that reflect everyone's heritage and honor special individual skills. Ask the children involved to write down and then "test" the recipes of the older people. Throw a banquet to celebrate the combined culinary heritage of the group.

813
Start a life-drawing class
To interest people in the way real bodies look, start a life-drawing class at a venue in your community. Book models of different sexes, sizes, and at different life stages. This will encourage participants to start thinking about their perceptions of health, confidence, and body shape.

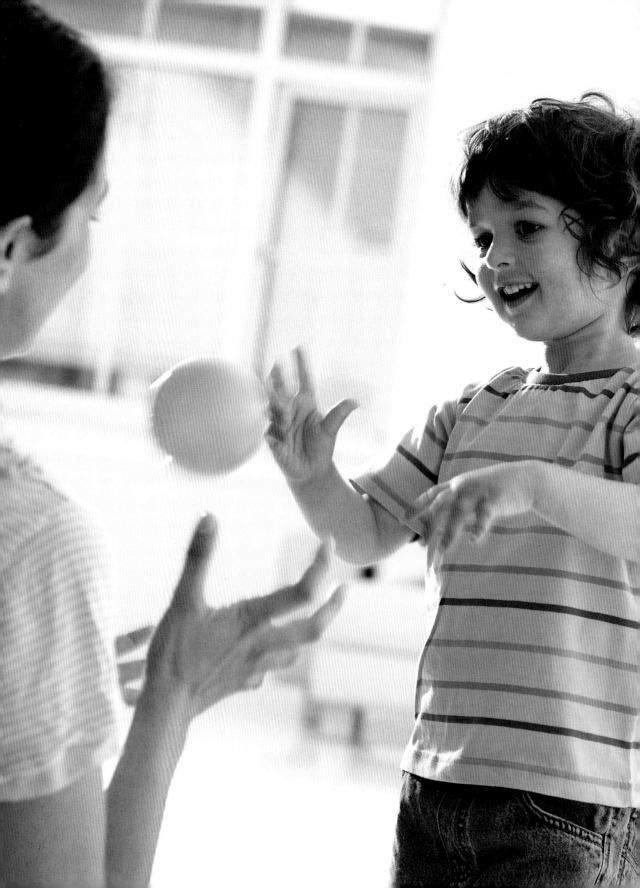

6 Family health fix

The eating and exercise habits we learn in childhood stay with us for the rest of our lives—so much so that maintaining a healthy weight in childhood reduces the risk of becoming an overweight adult, states the US government. In this chapter, you will find strategies to encourage healthy eating and outdoor play from the early days to ensure your child scores high on quality of life surveys. These are also strategies to keep you active and engaged with your child, from walking and swimming with a baby to cooking and growing food with older children. This chapter doesn't neglect grandparents, either, because to keep in shape, you need to be more rather than less active as you move into each new decade.

Include your baby in your daily exercises, to make the routine more enjoyable.

Post-natal reshaping

Most women find the post-baby bulge hard to shift. It's especially difficult to lose weight in the early months, when you hardly have a moment for yourself and are overwhelmed with sleeplessness (there is a link between lack of sleep and weight gain). Here are some ways to get moving again.

814
Rest first

Wait six weeks after the birth before exercising or dieting. Focus first on rebuilding your strength and energy levels with healthy foods: lots of fruit and vegetables, whole grains and pulses, low-fat milk and yogurt, plus sources of iron such as red meat, chickpeas, or no more than two portions of oily fish a week. Drink plenty of water, and rest as much as you can.

815
Reshape your pelvic floor

Start this exercise the day after giving birth to tone your pelvic floor and help prevent stress incontinence. The exercise also boosts blood flow, helping to heal your perineum. Simply squeeze and lift the sling of muscles between your pelvic bone and the base of your spine, as if trying to stop yourself peeing. Hold for a few seconds, then relax. Don't clench your buttocks. Repeat

8 times. As you get used to the exercise, squeeze your pelvic floor in and out quickly for 10 seconds, or pull up and down in stages. Repeat as often as you remember.

816
Yogic energy visualization

Sit comfortably with your spine upright, close your eyes, and pull up your pelvic floor muscles. As you inhale, visualize energy from your pelvic region flowing up your spine; as you exhale, feel energy spilling out around your heart and warming the center of your chest. Repeat for up to 1 minute.

817
Homeopathic repair

To help tone your perineal area, take the homeopathic remedy Sepia 30 daily for a few days to accompany your pelvic floor exercises. Consult a homeopath for treatment to help you recover physically and emotionally from giving birth.

818

Slim expectations

Be realistic; only celebrities with personal trainers are back in skinny jeans days after giving birth. You'll probably need your pregnancy waistbands for a while and an even bigger bra if you plan to breastfeed.

819

Breastfeeding benefits

Mothers who breastfeed exclusively for the first few months after giving birth tend to lose 1lb (0.5kg) a week—the target for healthy weight loss—without even trying. Breastfeeding helps protect your baby against childhood illnesses and allergies, and also gives your bones some protection from osteoporosis fractures later in life.

820

How many more calories?

Research suggests that for the first three months of breastfeeding, you need only around 300–400 calories a day on top of your recommended intake of 2,000 calories. That's a banana, a slice of whole grain bread with butter, and a glass of skim milk.

821

Timing is all

Cultivate patience and understand that it may take 10–12 months to get back to your pre-pregnancy weight.

822

Body changes

Post-pregnancy, you may eventually return to the weight you once were, but not the same shape. Many of us find that our ribcage widens and feet lengthen, our breasts get larger or smaller, and no type or amount of exercise shifts that belt of saggy skin

823

Forward bend with baby

This not only tones the muscles in the back of your legs, back, and abdomen, it amuses your baby. Try to repeat daily, noticing how you can hold the pose for longer and descend deeper after a few weeks' practice.

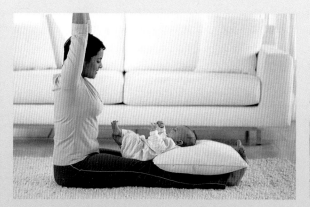

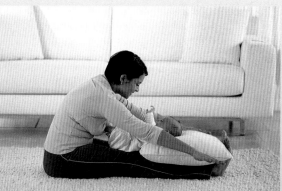

1 Sit with your legs outstretched and feet together. Place a cushion on your lower legs and your baby on the cushion. Sit up tall and stretch your arms overhead. Pull in your tummy muscles.

2 Exhaling, stretch forward, talking to your baby. Hinge from your hips (don't worry about getting too low). Try not to round your upper back. Hold the pose for a few moments. Return upright on an in-breath.

around the tummy. It's probably best to think of it as a well-earned badge of motherhood.

Take a walk

Walking is the easiest form of exercise in the post-natal months because you can take your baby with you: place her in a sling or a stroller that faces you, so she can see your face as you walk.

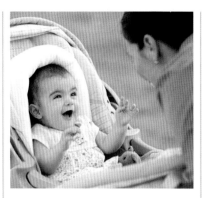

Take a walk with your baby. It's gentle exercise for you and fun for her.

825
Find a baby massage class

Take your baby out to a massage class where you can both socialize with other moms and babies. This can be particularly helpful if you suffer with baby blues (depression and obesity are linked).

826
Post-partum yoga

Look for a course that offers companionship as well as exercise, and introduces meditation techniques to help you through the early weeks when an active life seems a world away.

827
Take it easy

The hormone relaxin makes your joints extra loose during pregnancy (it encourages the ligaments in your pelvis and your cervix to relax in labor). The effects last for five or more months after birth, so to avoid injury, go easy when you exercise.

828
Baby press

To exercise your arms and the pectoral muscles in your chest, place your baby on the floor and adopt a push-up position with knees and feet on the ground. Bend your elbows to lower your upper body toward your baby, talking to her, then, breathing out, press on your palms to straighten your arms and lift you back to your starting position. Repeat 10–12 times.

829
Colorful fruit

Yellow and orange fruits and vegetables contain carotenoids and flavonoids that seem to promote a healthy immune system.

Try roasting winter vegetables—carrots, sweet potato, pumpkin, squash, beets—with rosemary, and serve with bacon.

830
Baby sit-up

To tone your abdominal muscles, lie on your back with knees bent and together, and feet flat on the floor. Place your baby on your lap, supported by your thighs. Lie back, head on the floor and arms crossed over your chest. Exhale, pull in your tummy muscles, sit up, and say "hello" to your baby. Inhale to lower with control. Repeat 10–12 times.

831
Check it out

If you put on a lot of weight during pregnancy and now can't lose it, your thyroid function may be out of balance. See your doctor for a check-up. You could also consult a homeopath for remedies to stimulate the thyroid.

Brightly colored peppers may help to boost your immunity.

Outdoors with a baby

Getting outdoors every day with your baby not only helps you to shed excess weight, it prevents cabin fever. Isolation is one of the key barriers to keeping in good mental shape during the early months of parenthood. You can also introduce your baby to the great green world. Establishing a habit of outdoor activity early in life influences health into old age.

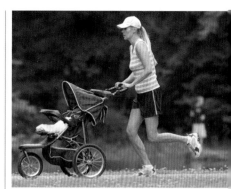

Build up fitness by jogging with the stroller—it gets you and your baby outdoors.

832
Start a walking group

Arrange to meet other mothers or grandparents with babies in strollers once or twice a week to walk to a baby-friendly café or gallery, or around a park. Look for hills to push up! Larger towns and cities often have baby-walking or stroller fitness groups you can join—look on the notice boards in specialist baby and health food stores.

833
Celebrate the seasons

Surveys suggest that children who have very early memories of nature tend to be more active outdoors as adults. They often also grow up to become the environmentalists of tomorrow, helping to keep our planet in shape. When out and about with your baby, introduce her to the changing seasons by allowing her to see, touch, and smell nature in the form of crunchy leaves, sticky buds, pussy willow, and hedgerow fruits.

834
Walk-run circuit

Slowly build up your walk with the stroller to a 15-minute jog and recovery-walk session. Walk for 5 minutes, then jog for 1 minute; walk for 4 minutes, then jog for 1 minute; walk for 3 minutes, then jog for a minute. Try to do this twice. After a few weeks, increase the amount of time you spend jogging and reduce the recovery walk until you can jog for 30 paces and walk for 30 paces. Be careful not to jolt your baby—try to stick to well-maintained paths.

835
Get your baby out

Babies are much more mobile than in the past, strapped into "travel systems" that allow you to move them without disturbance from car to supermarket cart to bedroom. Some pediatricians are concerned that an increase in cranial distortion, or flat-head syndrome, over the past decade may in part result from babies spending extended time in car and bouncy seats, infant carriers, and swings. To keep your baby's head well shaped and protect the spine from "lolling" injury, take her out of the car seat when you're not driving and wean her from sleeping in seats. Instead, carry her in your arms or a sling, sit her on your lap, or place her on her tummy (see No. 836).

836
Tummy time

Giving your baby "tummy time"—lying prone—when he's awake helps to prevent deformations of the skull and builds up strength in his upper shoulder girdle, which he needs for motor development. Give him a gentle back massage over his pajamas as he lies there, and place your head on the floor in front of him and talk to encourage him to lift his head. Always stay with a baby in the prone position.

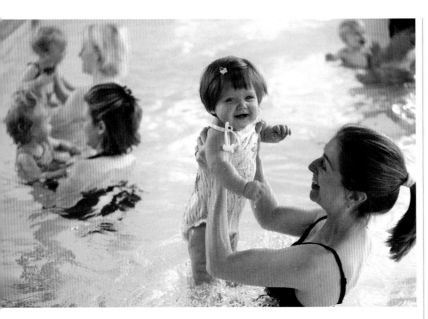

Babies and small children love water, especially if they are introduced to it when very young.

837
Try a bumbo seat

These colorful seats are designed for babies who can't yet sit unaided. They support the lower back, stabilize the pelvis, position the hip and knee joints to reduce strain on the spine, and help the baby practice trunk and head control. Bumbo seats are light enough to carry to cafés, parks, and friends' homes.

838
Sling benefits

Babies who spend time in slings tend to be calmer, more attached to their mothers, and cry less in the evening than babies who are kept in a seat. They may also develop better balance and muscle tone. You benefit, too, because using a sling puts less of a strain on your back and shoulders than carrying a car seat. Try different types of slings to find one that suits your stature as well as your baby's comfort. (Some researchers worry that vertical carriers that support a baby's weight only at the crotch can stress the spine.) Some slings can be adapted to allow a new baby to lie flat, an older baby to face forward or into your body, and a toddler to sit on your hip or back.

839
Little dippers

Swimming may improve babies' physical development and help them sleep and eat better than non-swimmers. Teach your baby to love the water by starting baby-swim classes from around 8–12 weeks. The fitness advantage for you is that you're expected to join the class. It's best to take a class with safety-certified baby-swim teachers, but you can practice between sessions. Make sure the water is warm enough: at least 90°F (32°C) for babies under 12 weeks and 86°F (30°C) for older babies. Sessions of 10–30 minutes are long enough.

840
Brain movement

Getting your baby moving in his first months with massage, baby yoga, and swim classes may increase his brain development. Babies move with most ease in the weightless environment of water. If you can't get to a baby-swim class, boost your infant's body awareness and have fun by playing together in the bath.

841
Practice at home

To practice water skills in the bath, get in with your baby and move her through the water on her back (keeping her head and shoulders well supported). Pour a little water over her head and face, and once she can sit up, practice blowing bubbles at each other. Also let her play with bowls of water in the kitchen and garden (always stay in attendance when a baby is near water).

Life with lively toddlers

It's hard to keep up with a busy toddler, but try to resist the temptation to get a break by putting him in front of the TV. Other than when your child is asleep, he should not be sedentary for longer than an hour. Luckily, playing with a lively toddler is a great way of working off stubborn post-baby weight.

842
How much activity?
For toddlers, experts recommend at least 30 minutes a day of structured physical activity and 60 minutes to several hours of free physical play. As your child nears preschool age (3–5 years), he needs at least 60 minutes of structured physical activity a day and several hours of unstructured physical play.

843
Be a role model
Toddlers like to copy what you and other family members do. Let them see you turn off the TV and go out on a bike, kick a ball around, or put on a wetsuit and go surfing.

844
Teach your child to catch
Children who fail to develop fundamental movement skills early in life become three times more sedentary than children who do acquire those skills. To introduce throwing and catching skills to your toddler, don't play just with balls, which can be hard to catch, use beanbags and soft toys as well.

845
Catch your shadow
On sunny days, play shadow games. Can you run away from your shadow, make it bigger and smaller, walk backward, or join someone else's shadow?

846
Coordination rhymes
Help your toddler's brain and language skills coordinate with body movement by singing body rhymes, such as, "I kick with my right foot, right foot, right foot; I kick with my right foot, just like this."

847
Fit and fun
Organized toddler fitness-fun sessions offer structured physical activity in well-thought-out circuits.

These provide opportunities to master "physical literacy" skills through play and to learn social skills such as sharing, cooperating, and listening to instructions.

848
Mommy and me clubs
Rather than sitting and reading a magazine while your toddler jumps in a ball pond, find a place where you can join in, too. Try toddler gyms, where you learn basic rolls, tumbling, balance, and coordination skills alongside your child.

849
Baby music sessions
Although these types of sessions are advertised as music-based, they all involve dancing and action songs,

Get outdoors and kick a ball around. Your toddler will soon want to join in.

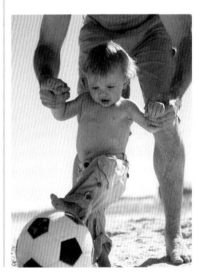

marching, lifting, and jumping as well as fostering the fine-motor skills needed to play hand-held percussion instruments.

850

Dance like an animal

At home, put on different types of music and dance with your toddler. Find music that makes you move like an elephant, a mouse, and a bird.

851

Fast and slow

Alternate activities at home, following fast-paced movement with slower activities to avoid over-winding your child.

852

Animal yoga

Do these movements together in a continuous sequence.

Downward Dog: start on hands and knees, then push your bottom up in the air and press back with your hands. Bark three times, then return to hands and knees or try to walk around on hands and feet.

Cobra: lie on your tummy, place your hands under your shoulders and straighten your arms to arch backward. Then lie flat again and wriggle like a snake, hissing.

Butterfly: sit with the soles of your feet together then flap your knees up and down like wings.

853

Making the team?

Don't pressurize your child to join a formal sports team or take organized sports-technique lessons until he or she is at least six years old. Below this age, children learn best through unstructured play.

854

Leave that child alone

Make space in the day for children to do their own thing—to play in an unstructured way without adult interference. This promotes brain development, creativity, and leadership and cooperation skills.

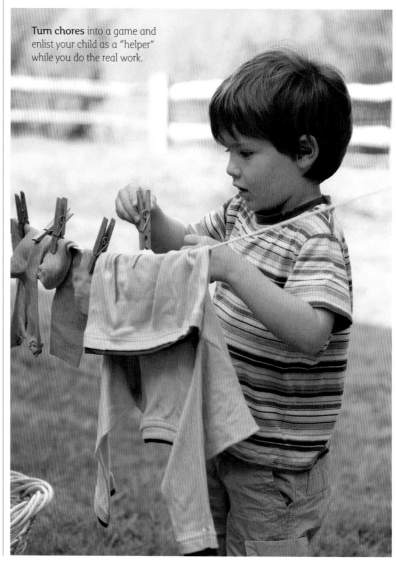

Turn chores into a game and enlist your child as a "helper" while you do the real work.

855
Home help

If you're easily bored by toddler games, have your child "help" you as you stay active around the home—sorting and hanging laundry, sweeping the floor, scrubbing the bathroom, and putting away groceries.

856
Getting the right balance

Fruits and vegetables are good for your child—but too much fiber can prevent adequate nutrient intake. Children under five also need calories and fats to grow properly. Make sure your child gets cheese, yogurt, butter, and whole milk daily, and choose mostly white bread, cereals, and pasta. Toddlers also need red meat and fish daily.

857
Snack-time

Toddlers have small tummies and need frequent snacks to stay in a good mood and have enough energy to be active. Try these:
- Fruit muffin
- Carrot cake
- Small box of raisins
- Small banana
- Satsuma
- Handful of cornflakes
- Yogurt
- Bread sticks with a hummus or soft cheese dip

Winding down

It is important to teach babies and children that while the daytime is for physical activity, the evening is for winding down, and nighttime is for sleeping. As various studies have shown, the connection between regular loss of sleep and an increased risk of obesity seems to be particularly significant in children.

858
Crack children's sleep

Follow a routine every night. After a quiet playtime, bath, milk, brushing teeth, and a story, put your child in bed while she's awake (but drowsy).

859
Buy new curtains

If you can still see the room when you put out the light, change or line your child's curtains, or fit blackout roller blinds.

860
Dark and quiet

For instant peace (especially with more than one child), draw the curtains in the bedroom, switch off

Make calming chamomile tea at bedtime.

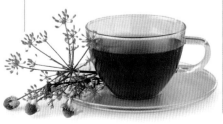

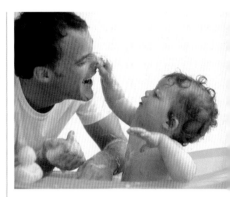

Make bathtime part of your child's evening routine, leading on to story time, then bed.

glaring overhead lights (keep one low light in a corner), and ask the children to tip-toe in using gestures and whispers. Then you can begin a quiet story or lullaby.

861
Tea ritual

Chamomile flowers contain a mild natural sedative. Make a bedtime ritual out of drinking chamomile tea with restless children who find it hard to wind down at bedtime. If you have space, grow and dry the flowers (German chamomile, *Matricaria recutita*). Pour 1 cup of boiling water over 1 tsp dried flowers, steep for 10–15 minutes, strain, and add honey for a treat. Limit children to ½ cup per day.

862
Massage your child
A number of studies have found that following a bedtime massage, infants and preschool children fall asleep more easily and quickly and sleep for longer. They may also be better behaved when awake. Try to start young, before they can crawl or run away. See the technique given below for a hand and foot massage.

863
Rhyme time
If your toddler doesn't tolerate being massaged, he may enjoy rhyming play with his hands and feet. A traditional rhyme names each finger or toe in turn and might keep him interested. Try "This little piggy went to the market..."

864
Calming busy children
Very busy children may benefit enormously from constitutional homeopathic treatment, as can their parents, particularly if the children's behavior veers toward the reckless or destructive.

865
Calming foods
To calm restless behavior in children, try introducing more of the following foods into their daily diet, which are high in vitamin B6: sweet potatoes, chickpeas, bananas, and fish. Vitamin B6 is required by the body for the synthesis of the neurotransmitter serotonin, which helps to regulate not only moods and emotions, but appetite and sleep.

866
Hand or foot massage
To get an older child accustomed to being massaged, begin with a hand. It may help to provide a distraction while you massage—perhaps some music or a story. When the child feels less ticklish, adapt the strokes for each foot.

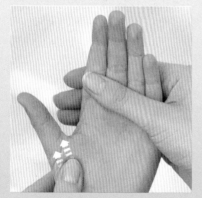

1 Rest the back of your child's hand in your fingers. Gently circle the palm with your thumb. Start small and gradually work outward.

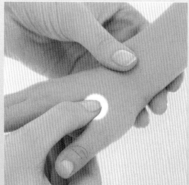

2 Repeat the circling movements over the back of the hand. Then trace the channels running from the wrist to the base of the fingers.

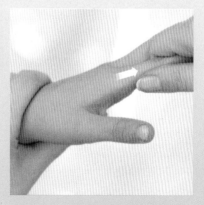

3 Roll each finger between your thumb and first finger, pressing the fingertip to finish. Then gently rub the hand between your palms.

Switching off

Time spent in front of a screen—TV, computer, or video game—correlates with childhood obesity. TV is also known to make children passive and slow the development of language skills. Harvard School of Public Health research suggests that the risk of being overweight is four times greater than average in children who watch more than five hours of TV daily.

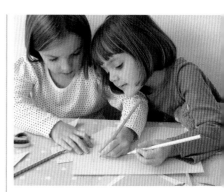

Play benefits your child more than the TV.

867
How much TV time?

Childcare experts advise that children under the age of two should never watch TV or DVDs. Older children should watch less than one or two hours a day. Parents are advised to monitor the programs.

868
Why turn off?

Turning off the TV may not encourage a child to exercise more, but it could still help weight loss. Children tend to consume more food and drink in front of a screen.

869
Commercial viewing

Exposure to TV ads for sugary, high-calorie, and nutrient-lite snacks and breakfast cereals is linked to obesity. When your child does watch TV, choose a channel with no advertising, or put on a DVD movie.

870
TV stops creativity

The more children watch television, the less likely they are to play imaginatively. But fantasy play helps children to acquire complex language skills, explore social roles, entertain themselves, and express emotions. Shape up your child for life by switching off.

871
Don't watch, talk

Children under 22 months don't learn words from children's TV programs. Talk to your infant to shape his language skills.

872
Play in and out

Outdoor play and TV watching aren't mutually exclusive. In a Canadian study of young people who play sedentary video games, 91 percent said they also enjoyed socializing outdoors.

873
Teens TV

TV viewing for teens is on the rise, particularly for teenage girls watching late at night or early in the morning. If your teens watch for hours, chat with them about the issues.

874
Monitor it

Keep the TV or computer in a family room so you know how long your child spends on it. Seeing family in the background of a web cam also deters online predators.

875
Ditch the babysitter

Children are so transfixed by TV that it seems to make life easier. But Yale University research found that viewing led to a shortened attention span, lack of reflectiveness, and expectation of rapid change. Finding time to play now can bring an easier life in the long run.

Active indoors

Children who are active are better achievers at school, have increased self-confidence, and reduced risk of suffering from depression or stress. They are also less likely to be overweight. Here are ways to keep children away from the TV when it's cold or rainy outside. And ways to keep you active, too.

876
Daily activity

Children aged from 6 to 12 years need at least 60 minutes and up to several hours of physical activity most days, advises the National Association for Sport and Physical Education in the US. This can be spread through the day—children shouldn't sit still for more than two hours at a stretch.

877
Hang a trapeze

Locate a beam in your living space, screw in hooks, and install a rope ladder, trapeze, or gym rings for kids to hang from when it's too wet to play outside. It's good for upper-body strength, coordination, balance, and self-confidence.

878
Runaround game

Get a pack of cards—for each suit allocate a room in your home; for each number allocate a letter of the alphabet (1 =A, 2=B, and so on). Shuffle the cards, place them in a pile on the floor, sit in a circle, and take turns to turn over a card. The suit tells you which room to run to, the

Turn up the music and create a home disco for your children and their friends.

number a letter of the alphabet. Run to that room and find something beginning with that letter, then run back with it. Set a timer for each run. Stay active after the game ends by taking everything back to its place.

879
Body tricks

Try this one with the kids. Stand in a doorway and stretch out your arms so that the backs of your wrists touch the doorframe on both sides.

Press your wrists into the frame and hold for one minute. Let go and walk forward. What happens to your arms?

880

Loaf sculptures

Buy one large white bread loaf per child and slice off the top. Ask children to scoop out and save the doughy insides. Then they can turn the hollow loaf into a vehicle or fantasy house by cutting windows, doors, and other features. Use the dough as modeling material to make figures and furniture, decorating it with pens, icing, or food-coloring.

881

Magic carpet yoga journey

Sit the children on a rug. Ask them to close their eyes and imagine they are flying to another land. When they land, ask them where they are. What can they hear, see, and smell? Ask them to open their eyes and take turns describing their country.

882

Home disco

Invite your children and their friends to work out dance routines to favorite tunes. Can they write a tune and lyrics and record it on the computer to dance to?

883

Body map

Get children to lie in turn on a big sheet of paper while a friend draws an outline around them to create a

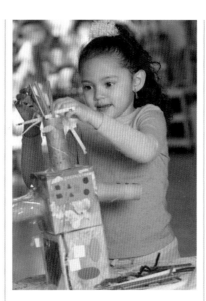

With a little imagination and a few bits of scrap, anyone can be an artist.

body map. Inside the body, ask them to write down the things that keep the body fit. Outside the body, record unhealthy things. By the head, write down ways of improving health, such as learning to cook.

884

Theater arts schools

Afterschool children's theater groups are a great way to promote body awareness and self-esteem by teaching dance and singing, as well as drama and improvisation.

885

Fun days at galleries

Art galleries and museums are fantastic places to keep fit if you follow an art trail along corridors

and spend time sitting on the floor to sketch. Look for art trolleys and explorer backpacks.

886

Scrapheap challenge

Host a group of kids and give them an afternoon challenge—perhaps to choose five recycled items to make into a boat that floats, or a windmill, or lighthouse. Look at a children's science book for ideas. Using the brain and their large and fine motor skills keeps bored children in shape.

887

Become a photographer

Give your child a challenge to produce a portfolio of photographs on a theme—perhaps food, friends, or wildlife. Encourage your child to look at his subjects from various angles—to crouch down, climb on a chair, get so close up that colors blur, or to move away so the subject is a tiny feature in a landscape.

888

What did grandma do?

Make a trip to see grandparents or elderly neighbors and ask them to describe the activities they enjoyed as a child. Write down what they say or record them on a dictaphone. See if your child can resurrect an old skipping game or rhyme, cycle trick, juggling feat, or magic act.

Children outdoors

Outdoor play in natural settings is especially important for children's development. Of course, it makes them more physically active, but also develops their intellect and leaves them feeling more emotionally and spiritually at ease. But in our eagerness to protect children from risk—traffic, strangers, other youngsters—we restrict their outdoor lives. Here are some safe outdoor activities to counter this trend.

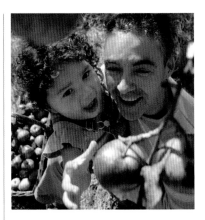

A special fruit tree of her very own will give your child an interest in being outdoors.

889
Getting dirty
In one study, 72 percent of children questioned said they avoided messy play because their parents dislike dirt. Get over your phobia, especially when children are young, to gear up your child for an active

Get your children out into the garden with a sunflower-growing competition.

future. Research shows that early oral exposure to microbes strengthens immunity and offers protection from allergic disorders.

890
Count the blades
Ask your child to lie on the grass to look for bugs or count the blades. Then get her to look up into the sky. What can she see, smell, and feel?

891
Make a daisy chain
Show your child how to make a daisy chain. Pick daisies with long stalks, slit the end of a stem with a thumbnail, and thread the next stem through.

892
Develop your front garden
Many front gardens have turned into a hardstanding for parking. A little effort can transform this space

into a green oasis that encourages children to get outside. Plant a hedge or cover the tarmac with pot plants that your child can look after.

893
Sunflower competition
See who can grow the tallest sunflower. Choose a giant variety and sow one seed per small pot of potting compost. Transplant to a sunny position when the stalks are 3in (7cm) tall. Water regularly. After flowering, hang up the heads to dry, then toast the seeds for snacking.

894
Plant a fruit tree
Plant a tree to mark a child's first birthday and to entice him outdoors to picnic beneath the blossom, climb the branches, rake up dead leaves, and, best of all, eventually enjoy freshly picked fruit.

895
Woodland play
Studies from Scotland and Singapore show that the frequency with which children visit woodland is the single most important factor in how much time they spend in woodland as adults. Visit woods at special times, perhaps when the bluebells are out or when the leaves change color.

896
No camera day
Take a child to a special place without his camera or phone so he has to engage at first hand rather than through a viewfinder.

897
Leave the car at home
Plan family trips to places of natural beauty and take the bus or train to get there. This gives your children the skills and confidence to travel on their own when they are older.

898
Get over the Grimms
We have long mythologized the forest as a dark place where children get lost or are lured into danger by strangers, but in fairy tales forests are also places where children defeat the witch and find sanctuary. Talk about this with your children to help them feel safe outdoors.

899
Adding value
Hook up a rope swing—in one study, children found woods with activities more fun than "just" trees.

900
Stalking skills
Practice moving in silence outdoors without anyone knowing you're there. To walk with no sound, bend your knees and land on the balls of your feet, making sure the ground is crackle-free before pressing your weight into your heel. Repeat over different types of terrain—on the beach, on pavement, in woodland. Be sure not to leave tracks.

901
Experiment outdoors
Do a science experiment outdoors: measure shadows at different times of day or make a glider and fly it. In a study by the California Department of Education, pupils following an outdoor science program improved their test results by 27 percent.

902
Green destressing
Stressed children may do better if they play in natural settings, says University of Illinois research. One hour a day spent in the natural world is thought to be helpful.

Woods are wonderful places for play and may help children feel less stressed.

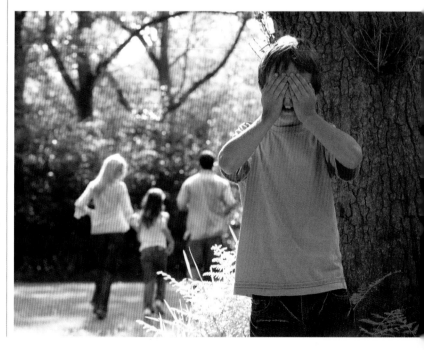

Kids outside alone

Playing outside unaccompanied encourages children to be responsible, improves social skills, and raises self-esteem. But what about their safety? Counter-intuitively, letting our children go makes them safer, because they learn to appraise risk and to make judgments that will help them survive in the wider world.

903
Be spontaneous

Child-led free outdoor play—with no obvious goal or adult direction— may be the only thing kids need to make them more active. University of London research found that all the walking and playing involved provided more exercise than most other activities.

904
Keep in good mental shape

Lack of time for free outdoor play is known to be a factor in the rise of mental illness in children and young people. Free play allows children to experience a range of emotions

Free play helps children to learn about themselves and the world around them.

including fear, anger, shock, pride, and sympathy. This shapes resilient human beings.

905
Building emotional health

Let your children have some secret, no-adults-allowed time outdoors in order to connect to the natural world. Campaigner Richard Louv suggests that lack of experience of nature leads to a tunneling of senses and a childhood marked by feelings of isolation and containment.

906
Clear your schedules

In 2004, England's Chief Medical Officer advised that children should have at least three or four play opportunities a week. Can you clear clubs and schoolwork to allow this?

907
Unofficial play spaces

Children value unplanned, marginal places away from the adult gaze over playgrounds and parks. Such places might include fields, barns, and woods, which offer scope and freedom for activities such as fort building. If your children do this, negotiate a set of safety rules.

908
Adventure playgrounds
Child-only playgrounds can feel safe for children and adults alike. If you can get your child involved in the design and build of a playground, they're more likely to find it a satisfying place to play and so stay active for longer.

909
Growing yourself
Letting children go out alone is how parents learn to trust in the face of uncertainty and become more confident. Reshape your values by welcoming the opportunity to grow and learn alongside your children.

910
Accepting risk
Children playing unsupervised outdoors inevitably face some risk. As parents, we need to weigh whether this risk poses more dangers than the risks to long-term physical, mental, and emotional well-being of being stuck indoors most of the time. Stay-at-homes are also not learning the skills that keep everyone safe in the outside world.

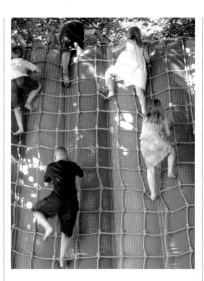

If an activity is fun, it stands to reason that your kids will want to keep on doing it.

911
Building a community
Get together with a group of parents and agree on a place and time to let the kids play on their own. You could start at a park, after setting meet-up points and pick-ups.

912
Give them a phone
Use technology for reassurance, and give your child a mobile phone. You can call to check up and he can get in touch in an emergency.

913
Ease into it
Camping trips to woods and wild places provide good opportunities to practice letting go. Encourage

children to build forts, look after younger siblings, and resolve arguments among themselves without coming back for adult help.

914
Letting go essences
The following flower essences may be helpful:
- Illawara Flame Tree: for the parent who experiences a child's growing independence as rejection.
- Yellow Cowslip Orchid: this helps you to be less controlling and negative.
- Dog Rose: for parents who torment themselves with "what if."

915
Grounding meditation
When you feel stressed about letting go, close your eyes and breathe in slowly, feeling a warm glow around your heart. As you breathe out, imagine the warmth traveling down your spine and then down through your buttocks or feet into the earth. Let go of your worries into this downward flow of energy.

916
Help them out
If your children can't play outdoors with other kids because transport is an issue, organize a roster of parents to ferry them to and from the woods, park, or swimming spot.

Reluctant teammates

Many children actively dislike organized or team games. Finding ways to tempt these children away from the screen or couch can be trying. Here are some ideas to help. Children who learn movement skills are likely to acquire more of the self-confidence needed to take part in sports, and so reduce their risk of obesity.

917
Learn to ride a bike

If your child is struggling to learn to ride a bike, don't use training wheels—they can delay her gaining balance skills. Try taking off the pedals and lowering the seat so her feet reach flat to the ground. She can push herself around, gradually lifting her feet higher.

918
Double dutch

Practice jumping rope at home to give your child the confidence to take part at school. Find two helpers to turn the rope while your child skips. Gradually turn the rope faster as he gains confidence.

919
Rhyming games

Help your child learn to skip to rhymes : those that have counting at the end allow you to compare scores with other jumpers. Try this one: "All in together girls, Very fine weather girls, When it's your birthday, All jump out: January, February, March," and so on.

920
Trampoline

Bouncing teaches balance, timing, and coordination skills, and improves muscle tone, bone mass, and circulation. Ten minutes of bouncing is said to be equivalent to a 30-minute jog or cycle ride. Choose a trampoline with a safety net, and allow only one child on it at a time.

Playing games with your child gives him the confidence he needs to play sports.

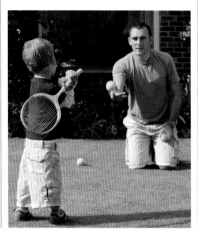

921
The novice skater

To lure a scared child into skateboarding, try downhill freestyling on a longboard. This is much larger than a regular board, so is more difficult to fall off, and they ride closer to the ground.

922
Garden Olympics

Set up a mini-Olympics circuit in your backyard, with "stations" for long- and high-jumping, a running track, and a wall for ball games. Offer prizes for whoever can bounce a ball or hula hoop the longest. End the day with a family relay race.

923
Show them how to stretch

Teach your children this easy post-sport stretch for the four main muscles in the legs: the quadriceps and hamstrings in the thigh and the gastrocnemius and soleus in the calf. It's good for easing tense, aching muscles after cycling and sports involving running.

Stand facing a wall with your knees together and left hand on the wall. Press your right heel to your right buttocks and hold, keeping your knees together.

Stand with your left foot near the wall and right foot behind you. Press your hands against the wall and feel a stretch all the way down the back of your thigh and calf.

Holding the position in the above step, bend your back knee until you feel a deeper calf stretch. Repeat everything on the other leg.

924
Sun Salutation sequence

This yoga sequence provides an activating stretch for the body's main muscles and is great for the whole family to learn.

Stand tall. Exhaling, bend forward and place your palms on the floor on either side of your feet. Step one foot back and then the other, pushing your buttocks toward the sky to make a mountain shape.

Without moving your hands, drop to your knees, then stretch forward along the floor (again without moving your hands or feet). When your shoulders are over your hands, push up, arching your back. **Push back** into the mountain shape, then step first one foot, then the other forward so you are in a standing forward bend. Inhale and stand back upright. Repeat all the steps, alternating which foot you step back with first. Repeat 6 times.

925
Try fit camp

Encourage children who feel limited by their body to try a fit camp. Fit camps are staffed by nutritionists, personal trainers, and counselors who make physical activity fun—and teach kids how to enjoy good food, too.

926
Support your teen

For the teenager who feels awkward and self-conscious in her rapidly changing body, look to female-only sports clubs or summer camps, where she might feel less stressed wearing sports gear and a bathing suit. These may also have a focus on raising self-esteem, which can give your daughter the confidence to take part.

Bounce to fitness on a trampoline. Your child will enjoy the sense of weightlessness.

The young gourmet

If children grow up enjoying a wide range of healthy foods, including plenty of fruits and vegetables, pulses, and grains, they are more likely to follow a good diet in adulthood. In particular, this equips them to avoid junk food in their teen and college years. It reminds you to eat properly, too.

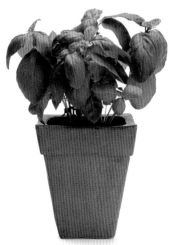

Teach your child to grow basil and use it to show him how fragrant food can be.

927
Learn to shop
Take your child on shopping trips and explain how to recognize the healthiest food. Compare labels on packets to spot hidden sugars (see No. 254) and invisible fruit (see tip 257), and try to spot foods containing whole grains.

928
Sodas
Keep your child from reaching into the refrigerator for sodas by talking to him about what's in them. A typical can of soda contains more than 8 tsp of sugar.

929
Drink aware
Teach kids to ignore the images and claims like "sugar-free" on juices and drinks, and to look for the key words on the label. Pure apple juice is just called "apple juice"; if it has added water and sweeteners, the label will say "apple juice drink."

930
Provide water
Keep a jug of water on hand throughout the day for active children to help themselves from. An extra soda daily increases a child's risk of obesity by 60 percent.

931
Take the taste test
Play the blindfold game: offer a child a sip each of orange juice from concentrate, freshly squeezed juice, orange juice "drink" containing sugar or sweeteners, and a can of orange soda. Ask him to describe the flavors and think about sweetness, bitterness, smell, and texture. Can he taste the difference between fresh and processed products? (The WHO blames obesity on the latter.)

932
Fruit fun
Buy lots of different fruit for younger kids. Cut up the larger fruits and wash the small berries.

Get a large tray or plate and make a fantasy fruit face or picture before eating it.

933
Taste poetry
Buy a pack of fridge-magnet poetry words and give your child a new food to taste—fruit, vegetables, salad leaf, or herb. Ask her to put together words that describe the taste and texture, and then use them to write a poem on the fridge.

934
Yum Yum Yuck
Melt some chocolate or carob drops and pour into ice cube molds. In one or two molds, place something edible but unexpected: an olive, clove of garlic, anchovy, or clove, then let set. Then play taste roulette with your children.

935
Find a barn

Type your zip code into www. localharvest.org to see a map of your local food producers, from bakeries to cheesemakers and oyster farms.

936
Grow basil

Show your toddler how to grow a thicket of basil by sowing a few seeds in a large pot of compost according to the packet instructions. Water, and keep on a sunny window sill or in a greenhouse. Growing things is a great way to get a child enthused about how fragrant and flavor-packed fresh food can be.

937
Shelling peas

Grow your own peas and beans for kids to pick and shell, providing another example of the intense pleasure hit of fresh seasonal food.

938
Cooking together

Even if your child is too young to be of any real help in the kitchen, encourage him to "cook" alongside you. Kids who handle real ingredients often learn instinctively what tastes good with what.

939
Cook your own lunch

Ask older children to help you cook a dish for their lunchbox, encouraging them to taste as they go along to help develop their palate. Cook up some tasty rice (basmati, brown, or wild) and mix in chopped fresh peppers, scallions, tomato, and cooked chicken. Or boil some pasta, then stir in tuna and corn.

940
Pick your own tomatoes

Lycopene is a plant nutrient that keeps the heart, eyes, and skin in good shape from the early years into old age. Tomatoes are the best source, and home-grown, still warm from the sun, the most delicious way to indulge.

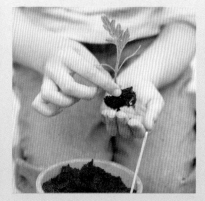

1 Scatter a few tomato seeds into an egg carton filled with potting compost, and cover them with a thin layer of compost. Water carefully.

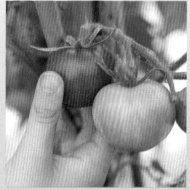

2 Transplant seedlings into separate pots. Plant into a grow-bag or large planter once flowers appear. Tie to a support cane.

3 Pinch out the plant top and any side shoots after five branches have formed. Water regularly, and feed weekly with tomato fertilizer.

941
Tortilla roll

Ask your toddler to choose the filling for a tortilla: ham, cheese, eggs, tuna, shredded lettuce, cucumber, tomatoes. Let him do the rolling up.

942
Calcium time

It's important that children get enough calcium, especially as they head into the teenage years: between the ages of two and eight they need two cups of milk daily; over the age of eight, three cups. Experiment with how much milk you can pour into smoothies, pancakes, and puddings.

943
Rice pudding

A toddler can help you make this. Place ½ cup short-grain pudding rice and 1 quart (1 liter) of warm milk in a saucepan. Add 2 tbsp sugar, a few pitted prunes, and 1 tbsp of butter, in pieces. Cook at 300°F (150°C), uncovered, for 2 hours.

Planning and cooking meals together gets the whole family interested in good food.

944
Milky popsicles

Pour low-fat drinking yogurt into paper cups, add a popsicle stick, and freeze until solid—peel off the cup before eating. For interest, add slices of strawberries or diced peach.

945
Your turn tonight

Everyone becomes more interested in good food if you plan what to eat together. Experiment with set meals for set days: burritos on Wednesday; homemade curry on Friday; roasted chicken with dessert for Sunday lunch.

946
Broadening an appetite

How many different types of food can you eat in a week? Start a competition in your home, getting children to make a food chart and tally up their scores.

947
ACE nutrients

Introduce good sources of the immunity-boosting vitamins A, C, and E to children early on, to ensure they keep eating them into adulthood. Find A and C in bright orange vegetables and fruits, tomatoes, red peppers, and dark leafy greens. Vitamin E is found in nuts and sunflower seeds and their oils.

Fussy eating

It's frustrating to invest effort, love, and precious time into creating healthy, home-cooked dishes only to have kids grumble or refuse to try a mouthful. Here are ways to avoid conflict and make meals less of an emotional battleground for everyone. Good eating habits start with babies' first solid food.

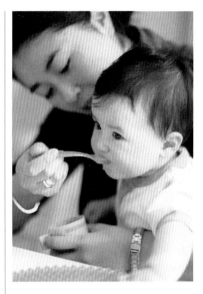

Babies weaned onto fresh foods are often less picky about new tastes as they get older.

948
What they like
In a study of infant and toddler food preferences, babies generally preferred purées while toddlers favored chunky-textured food. However, when babies in the study were given more complex textures to sample, they too preferred them. So start giving "proper" food from the outset as well as purées.

949
Baby-centered weaning
This is the art of moving infants directly from milk (after the age of six months) on to "real" food—

Think about texture as well as taste when you are tempting your baby to eat.

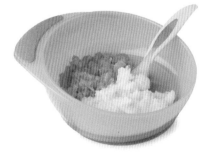

chunks of the home-cooked food you eat, rather than purée. At six months, babies have a greater ability to "chew" and swallow, and have sufficient hand–eye coordination for choosing and picking up food. Babies who go straight to the taste and texture of "real" foods (rather than processed jars) tend to be less picky about new tastes.

950
Chunk it up
The secret of successful baby-led weaning is to cut food into fist- or chip-sized chunks for easy grasping. Introduce cooked vegetables before fruit, so that babies don't get fixated on sweet tastes. Try steamed broccoli or carrots, baked sweet potato, grilled asparagus, or ripe avocado. Don't start to give starchy foods, fats, or protein-rich foods until 8–9 months.

951
Prepare for a mess
Baby-led weaning is messier than spooning purées into his mouth,

then wiping him clean between mouthfuls. Place newspaper beneath the high chair and buy huge bibs.

952
Eat with your infant
Make baby feeding time an occasion to sit and eat with your child. Even if you're not ready for a full meal, make a snack of something he is eating. This can seem like a chore, but is less so than having an 11-year-old who won't try "adult" food.

953
Ingredient watch
Try to avoid the following bulking ingredients in commercial baby foods: water; thickeners such as flour, tapioca, or corn starch;

sweeteners such as sugar and corn syrup. Foods containing these have been found to have less than 50 percent of the nutrients of those made with more fruit and vegetables.

954
Which jar?
When choosing one-ingredient babyfood jars, choose the one with most calories or carbohydrate content. It will also have the most fruit or vegetables—nutrients.

955
Make your own
Avoid jars of processed pudding completely—instead, mash a banana or soaked dried organic apricots and stir into full-fat natural yogurt.

956
Boycott toddler foods
Relying on processed baby food promotes the idea that children need separate food. This rapidly leads to buying dinosaur-shaped "toddler dinners" and cooking separate child and adult meals. Don't let your mealtimes be this complicated—or expensive.

957
Don't give up
Have courage and persistence— rather than serving your fussy eater

only the things she *will* eat. Eat as a family and serve everyone from the same dish. After a few hair-tearing weeks, she'll start eating most of it.

958
Snack time
Children—especially under the age of five— need snacks, since it's hard for their small tummies to take in enough nutrients and calories at one meal to keep them going until the next. However, many parents worry

that constant snacking disturbs mealtimes. Rather than putting out food to pick at all day, stick to set snack times—mid-morning and afternoon, and before bed.

959
Child-sized portions
A Penn State research study found that three-year-olds won't overeat, no matter how much food you pile on their plates. By the age of five, this changes: older children (like

Children and vegetables don't always mix. Stay calm and keep serving up the greens.

adults) will eat even when sated, if you keep giving them food. Reassess plate and portion sizes once your child nears school-age.

960
Freeze leftovers

If your delicious meals tend to be rejected, serve up only a small portion to start with and freeze the rest (in equally small portions).

961
Vegetable challenge

One mother tried everything to get her seven-year-old to eat more vegetables—treats, bribes, and battles. How did she get over it in the end? By challenging him to an online vegetable adventure to eat his way through an A–Z of vegetables, from asparagus to vegetable kebabs, with recipes posted from people around the world. Mom cooks and son Freddie eats, scores out of 10, and feeds back to those who suggested the ideas. Follow the adventure and contribute a recipe at www. greatbigvegchallenge.blogspot.com.

962
Watch your stance

How do you deliver food to the table? Do you thrust your face forward aggressively when serving up new dishes or food you know the kids dislike? Do you sigh and slump,

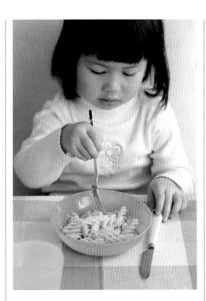

Let your child take her time with meals and don't fuss if she doesn't clear her plate.

projecting lack of confidence? Try bringing your shoulders back over your hips and your hips over your ankles; as you exhale, drop your shoulders and broaden your collarbones. This conveys a sense of calm and confidence.

963
Stop staring

Try not to scrutinize your child as she eats. In a study of female college students, the following early mealtime experiences were linked with bulimia nervosa: parents who dominated conversation; hostility; pressure to clean the plate and finish dinner at the same time as everyone else; food being used as punishment; food offered as a treat or to console a child who was upset.

964
Don't cry

If it really hurts when your children reject a lovingly prepared meal, take a few drops of Bach Flower Rescue Remedy to help you deal with the feelings without getting angry. The Australian Bush Essence Boab is useful if you notice a mealtime-behavior pattern repeating from your own childhood.

965
Seek a consultation

If you tend to be picky about food, your child may echo your behavior. Seek homeopathic treatment yourself if you have a capricious appetite or specific food likes and dislikes—you may respond well to a particular remedy.

966
Invite a friend

Research shows that children as young as two learn food preferences from their peer group, and so are more likely to try different foods if they see friends doing so. Make the most of this by inviting one or more of your child's friends who eat a variety of foods to share lunch. Try not to serve food you know your child will eat—this is the day of the week you can all be more adventurous.

Eating together

The good news? Children of families who eat together eat less fussily and more healthily—forever. The bad news? Children who don't eat regular meals with their family (and do watch TV) are more likely to be overweight, according to a 2008 study published in the *Journal of the American Dietetic Association.*

967
Turn off at dinner time
Most US families watch TV during dinner, found the National Institute on Media and the Family back in 1999; more than half of children in the UK now do the same. Be aware that this results in increased intake of food and calories.

968
Get everyone involved
Shared mealtimes work best if everyone—even the youngest member of the family—has a task, whether shopping, cooking, setting the table, or cleaning up.

969
Eat with your daughters
Regular family meals may offer some protection against eating disorders. A 1999 University of Minnesota survey found that teenage girls who ate five or more structured meals with their families each week were less likely, five years later, to use "disordered eating behaviors," such as vomiting and diuretics, to control their weight.

970
Eat breakfast
Working hours in families are so mismatched that breakfast may be

Involve the whole family at mealtimes by giving everyone a special task.

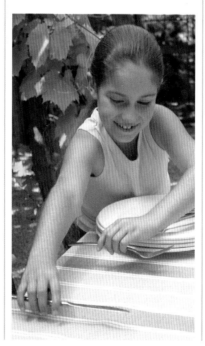

one of the few times we can eat together. Make this your incentive to wake everyone a half hour earlier.

971
Breakfast with teens
Research shows that young adults who skipped breakfast were unlikely to meet even two-thirds of their recommended daily intake of vital vitamins and minerals. Those who eat breakfast tend to be safe-guarded from substance abuse, antisocial behavior, and eating disorders.

972
Enjoy teen spirit
Persevere with surly teens at mealtime. Teens who eat family meals five days a week are reported to be less likely to take drugs or be depressed, are more motivated at school, and have better peer relationships than those who eat family meals only three days a week.

973
Keep it up
A University of Minnesota study found that eating as a family through adolescence set eating patterns that lasted. Young adults who shared family meals tended to eat more fruits and vegetables (getting significantly higher intakes of vitamins, minerals, and fiber) and drink fewer soft drinks.

974
Girls need calcium
If your girls hate calcium-building milk, plan family meals around calcium-rich alternatives: sardines and salmon; almonds and sesame seeds; and green leafy veggies, such as bok choy, kale, and broccoli.

975
Special time
Mealtime with toddlers can be a nightmare, but take heart. In a "family dinner experiment" on *Oprah*, families who ate together every night for a month kept a diary of their feelings. These diaries revealed how the children treasured family meals.

976
Flower Essences to keep anger at bay
Keep anger at bay around the table with these remedies:
• Snapdragon (Californian Flower Essence): when you'd like to be less snappy and verbally aggressive.
• Holly (Bach Flower Remedy): when your prickliness comes from a sense of hurt.

977
Talking in turn
Use mealtimes as an opportunity to talk around the table. Preschoolers

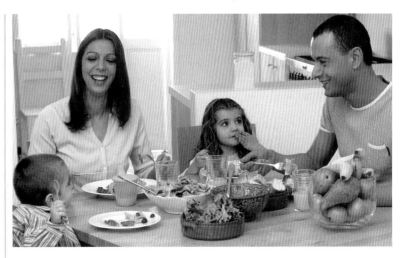

Shared meals are good opportunities for practicing manners and teaching language skills.

who eat with their families have better language skills and vocabularies because they are exposed to extended conservations.

978
Talking game
Play a game in which each person describes their favorite activity of the week, what made them laugh today, or the plot of a book. Or contribute one word each to a sentence around the table.

Broccoli is an excellent source of calcium, essential for healthy teeth and bones.

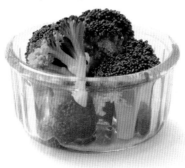

979
Share food memories
Sharing meals that are important to your food culture, and telling stories about how your ancestors ate raises children's self-esteem.

980
Knife and fork
Teach your preschool child to use a knife and fork. Get him to practice spreading butter, cutting and spearing, and swirling spaghetti.

981
Table manners
Modeling table manners is the best teaching tool: don't start eating until everyone has been served; stay seated until everyone has finished; give new dishes a try; and don't talk with your mouth full.

Lively children's parties

Parties are a license for eating fun foods, but they don't all have to be unhealthy. Serve some of these ideas alongside the chocolate and chips—and try out some of the ideas for games, too. To keep children extra active, have them help you prepare some of the lemonade and punches, chop up fruit and vegetables, and assemble the party bags.

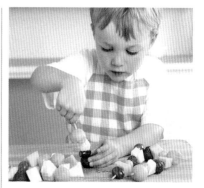

Making fruit kebabs is a great way of amusing children at a party.

982
Pink fruit punch
Mix together equal portions of cranberry juice and sparkling water. Add chopped strawberries, orange slices, and whole raspberries. Scatter a few mint leaves over the top.

983
Berry shake
For a filling energy drink at the start of a party to keep young guests away from the food table, use a blender or food processor to blend 1 pint each of strawberries and blueberries or blackberries with 6 tbsp plain yogurt and 2 cups cold milk. Serve garnished with chopped strawberries.

984
Lemonade
This is so much tastier than store-bought lemonade, and contains no sweeteners, flavorings, or additives.

4 lemons, unwaxed
4–6 tbsp superfine sugar, to taste
4 cups sparkling water, chilled
handful fresh mint leaves
lemon slices, to garnish

Remove the lemon zest with a vegetable peeler and place in a large jug. Squeeze the lemons and pour the juice and any pulp into the jug. **Add the sugar** and 1 cup boiling water and stir well until dissolved. Let cool, then refrigerate. **Add the sparkling water,** and garnish with the mint leaves and lemon slices. Serve over ice.

985
Stripey sandwiches
Make sandwiches from both white and whole grain bread, and arrange them alternately on a serving plate. You could also warm up whole wheat and white pita bread and cut it into strips for scooping up cream-cheese dips (add some chopped chives) or hummus.

 Sandwiches look more inviting when arranged in "stripes" of white and whole grain bread.

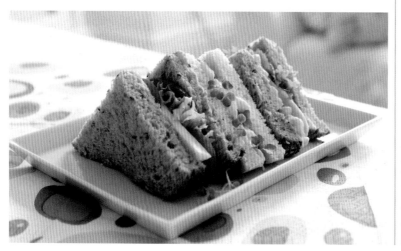

986
Top vegetables for parties
- Olives
- Cucumber or celery sticks
- Radishes
- Cherry tomatoes
- Chick peas
- Sliced red pepper
- Snow peas

987
Fruit and nut dip
Melt some 70 percent cocoa-solid chocolate and some white chocolate. Place in separate bowls and offer children cut-up fruit and large nuts—strawberries, kiwi, Brazil nuts, and cashews work well—to dip in the chocolate. Leave the dipped goodies to set on baking parchment.

988
Party taste test
Blindfold children and ask them to smell (or taste) and identify the following foods: lemon quarters, orange zest, mint leaves, chives, cocoa powder, coffee beans, honey, Marmite, marzipan, cloves, fennel, and blackcurrants.

989
Bobbing for apples
A great energetic food game. Place one apple per child in a big tub of water, tie back hair and put on plastic aprons, then ask guests to catch an apple with their teeth.

990
Fruit kebabs
Prepare bowls of grapes, diced pineapple and apple, melon balls, orange segments, and berries. Give each child a wooden skewer to thread with fruit. When everyone has finished, offer dips for dunking.

991
Top party fruit
- Pineapple chunks
- Watermelon
- Strawberries
- Blueberries
- Dried apricots or cranberries
- Raisins
- Seedless grapes.

992
Better chips
Choose unsalted chips that come with their own bag of salt. Popcorn is a good substitute. Add a little sea salt, or sweeten with a sprinkle of sugar or a drizzle of honey.

993
Party in a tree
Look for companies that run active children's parties: in a tree, in a drama studio, at a watersports venue or climbing wall, in the woods, or at the pool or skating rink. Or hire a hall and an active party entertainer: perhaps a cheerleader, sports coach, or circus-skills troupe.

994
Sports day party
Meet in a park and set up a series of fun races: sack race, three-legged race, dressing-up race, running backward race, egg (or ball) and spoon race, and a few relays.

995
Active parcel
Wrap up a gift, then pack it in layers of wrapping paper. In each layer hide a "forfeit"—a piece of paper detailing activities a child must do, such as a cartwheel, forward roll, standing on one leg for a minute, or hopping. Sit the children in a circle

Play pass the parcel and make sure all the forfeits involve some type of activity.

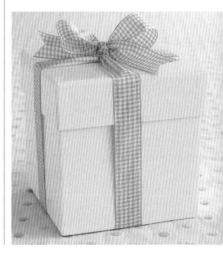

and pass around the parcel to music. When the music stops, the person holding the parcel takes off a layer and does the activity.

996
Musical games

What's a party without a good selection of musical games? Try musical chairs, statues, chairs or cushion, and a dancing competition.

997
Balloon games

See who can keep a balloon in the air for longest using only their head. Then get into teams to pass a balloon from person

For an active end to a party, get everyone to take turns hitting a piñata.

to person using no hands—wedge it between head and shoulder, or, for the more accomplished, start in pairs with a balloon lodged between chests.

998
Customize an apron

Buy one plain apron per child and plenty of fabric pens. Have ready some images from food magazines

to inspire the children. Ask each child to decorate his or her apron with the theme of food and chefs.

999
Party favors

For an active end to the party, put some a goodies in a piñata for the children to break open. If you prefer sugar-free gifts, try the following:

- Toothbrush
- Chinese jump rope
- Glow sticks
- Balloons
- Kite-making or glider kit
- Water pistols
- Small bouncy balls
- Bubbles

1000
Make your own bags

Make your kids get active and creative if they want to give away bags at the end of a party. Paint sheets of newspaper or plain brown paper according to a theme (sealife, space, butterflies, rainbow, glitter). Once the paper is dry, roll it into cones and secure with sticky tape. Then fill.

1001
Sleeping lions

A great game to end an active party. Players lie on the floor with their eyes closed pretending to be asleep. Those who move are out!

Resources

Good eating
www.bdaweightwise.com
www.eatright.org
www.eatwiththeseasons.com
www.shapeup.org
www.health.gov/
DietaryGuidelines
www.breakfastresearchinstitute.
org
www.localharvest.org
www.greatbigvegchallenge.
blogspot.com
www.michaelpollan.com

www.animalvegetablemiracle.com
joannasfood.blogspot.com

Getting active
www.bikeleague.org
www.cdc.gov/nccdphp/dnpa/
physical
www.arobuddhism.org
www.health.harvard.edu
www.osha.gov
www.realage.com
www.getintoreading.org
www.railtrails.org

www.spafinder.com
www.nwf.org
www.yogajournal.com
www.mapmyride.com
www.walktoschool.org.
www.kidsoutside.info
www.childrenandnature.org

Inspiring exercise books:
Yoga the Path to Holistic Health, B.K.S.
Iyengar (Dorling Kindersley 2007)
The Power of Breath, Swami
Saradananda (Duncan Baird 2009)

The New York City Ballet Workout
(Willam Morrow 2001)
Pilates Body in Motion, Alycea
Ungaro (Dorling Kindersley 2002)
*How You Stand, How You Move,
How You Live*, Missy Vineyard (an
introduction to the Alexander
Technique) (Da Capo Press 2007)
Zen in the Art of Archery, Eugen
Herrigel (Penguin 1988)
Last Child in the Woods, Richard
Louv (Algonquin Books of
Chapel Hill 2006)

Index

About the author

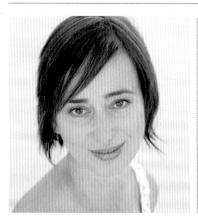

Susannah Marriott is a freelance writer who specializes in complementary healthcare. She is the author of 15 illustrated books on yoga, spa treatments, meditation and prayer, and natural approaches to pregnancy and parenting, including *1001 Ways to Stay Young Naturally*, *1001 Ways to Relax*, *Total Meditation*, *Basic Yoga*, *The Art of the Bath*, and *Your Non-Toxic Pregnancy*. Her writing has appeared in *Weekend Guardian* and *The Times*, *Zest*, *Top Santé*, *Healthy*, *She*, and *Marie Claire*, and she has broadcast on BBC Radio 4. Susannah lives with her husband and three young daughters in Cornwall, where she lectures on writing at University College Falmouth. She keeps in shape by practicing yoga, swimming in the Atlantic, camping, and growing her own fruits and vegetables.

Acknowledgments

Author's acknowledgments

Many thanks to everyone who gave me their healthy eating and exercise tips, especially all the WeightWatchers, Stephen Parker for suggesting and testing recipes, and my sea-swimming partner Rosie Hadden. Thanks to Mat Johnstone for foraging and cheesemaking advice, Hayley Spurway for coastal adventuring ideas, Jen Wight for climbing tips, and Paul Slydel at Cycle Solutions (01326 377003) for cycling advice. Special thanks to Julia Linfoot and Amanda Brown for their expertise; Peggy, Esther, and Helen at DK for their vision, and especially Angela and Carole for knocking everything into such great shape.

Contributors

Julia Linfoot BSc MCPH RSHom is a Registered Homeopath in practice in South London since 1999. She also prescribes herbal tinctures, flower essences, and tissue salts. She supervises student homeopaths and teaches courses in homeopathy and health.
Contact Bellenden Therapies on 0207 732 1417 or email juliahomeopath@btinternet.com

Amanda Brown has been teaching yoga for 20 years. She also practices as an artist and a natural therapist. Contact 01326 318776 or email magicbean_99@yahoo.co.uk

Publisher's acknowledgments

Dorling Kindersley would like to thank Alyson Silverwood for proofreading, Vanessa Bird for the index, and Ann Baggaley for editorial assistance. They would also like to thank Ruth Jenkinson for the new photography, Alli Williams for hair and make-up, and Rosie Hopper for styling. Thanks also to Suhel Ahmed and Sky Kang for their help with picture research. Lastly, thanks to our great models: Jo Freeman and Niki-Simone from Models Plus; Gail Shuttleworth from Model Plan; Kate Loustau and Heidi Cordell from Close Models; and Jas Kang, Susannah Marriott, and Charlotte Seymour.
Special thanks to MBT UK for the loan of their sandals (page 121).

31901050499146

Picture credits

The publisher would like to thank the following for their kind permission to reproduce their photographs:
(Key: b-bottom; l-left; t-top)

Alamy Images: DAJ 58t; Food & Beverages 97; Chuck Franklin 41b; Grain Belt Pictures 102-103; imagebroker 114t; Stan Kujawa 53; Photodisc 13; Tom Wood 52b; **Corbis**: Peter Adams/zefa 139; Artiga Photo 22t; Richard Baker/www.bakerpictures.com 153; Michael A. Keller 14t; Michael Keller 46; Steve Lupton 85t; Tom & Dee Ann McCarthy 137; Roy McMahon 50; Mika/zefa 100t; Jeffery Allan Salter 138; Brigitte Sporrer/zefa 54; **DK Images**: Courtesy of Simon Brown 182; **Getty Images**: Lori Adamski-Peek 21t; Peter Cade 172t; Tony Hopewell 133b; Clarissa Leahy 176; Ethan Meleg 150t; Microzoa 11t; Peter Nicholson 31; Bernd Opitz 124t; Tim Platt 11b; PM Images 87; Lisa Romerein 136l; Jed Share 10t; Juan Silva 128-129; Smith Collection 43; Paul Thomas 119; Luca Trovato 99b; **Photolibrary**: Awilli Awilli 111; Bananastock 16, 39, 75, 120t, 177; Blend Images 117b, 151, 171, 188; Botanica 101b; Corbis 14b, 55, 146-147, 162t, 165; Creatas 108, 163t; Denkou Images 26b; Digital Vision 12, 17t, 18t, 30, 33, 40, 49b, 56, 115, 117t, 118, 127, 143, 170, 184; Fancy 82t, 133t, 154t; Fogstock RF 8-9; image100 135, 140; Imagesource 42; IPS images 74b; Juice Images 157, 173; Juniors Bildarchiv 156; Kablonk! 145; Mauritius 122; Moodboard 65; Novastock 141; OJO Images 67; Paul Paul 174; Photoalto 88b; Photodisc 152; Polka Dot Images 64; H Schmid 103; Somos Images 83t; Stockbyte 45t, 63; Joakim Sundell 175; Thinkstock 128t; Uppercut Images 57, 116, 164; Westend 61 109; **PunchStock**: Digital Vision 18-19; Inspirestock 51; Radius Images 172b; **Red Cover**: Charlotte Murphy 59; **SuperStock**: age fotostock 91, 150b; Mauritius 86; Pixtal 88t; Prisma 124-125

All other images © Dorling Kindersley
For further information see: www.dkimages.com